Springer Biographies

The books published in the Springer Biographies tell of the life and work of scholars, innovators, and pioneers in all fields of learning and throughout the ages. Prominent scientists and philosophers will feature, but so too will lesser known personalities whose significant contributions deserve greater recognition and whose remarkable life stories will stir and motivate readers. Authored by historians and other academic writers, the volumes describe and analyse the main achievements of their subjects in manner accessible to nonspecialists, interweaving these with salient aspects of the protagonists' personal lives. Autobiographies and memoirs also fall into the scope of the series.

More information about this series at
http://www.springer.com/series/13617

Ian Howie

Reflections on a United Nations' Career

An Insider's Account

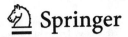

Ian Howie
Carlton, VIC, Australia

ISSN 2365-0613   ISSN 2365-0621   (electronic)
Springer Biographies
ISBN 978-3-030-77062-4   ISBN 978-3-030-77063-1   (eBook)
https://doi.org/10.1007/978-3-030-77063-1

Dedicated to Shoroni and Tim, who were on the journey, and to Mark who joined us later.

Foreword

This book was always going to be more than an autobiographical account of the career of a young man from Melbourne who spent his working life as a United Nations official. It is, in fact, a critical, indispensable debriefing of a UN insider's account as it follows the life of a development practitioner for more than three decades within the global aid sector.

It also goes where few others have dared to go before, providing first-hand insight into the realities of a UN career official's life. Whilst many throughout the world may wish to join the 'UN family' or have already become part of the development sector, it is presumed they all have a vision to act as vehicles for positive social change. However, expectations may differ once realities have sunk in. The book opens an important space in the international aid sector around elements of personal and professional rewards and costs.

What is it like to work for the UN? Why choose a career in the UN system? What do people actually do for the UN? Can a development practitioner really make a difference? As an outsider, how does one learn to navigate the ropes within the bureaucratic system? And, once in the system, what are the implications on family ties, relationships and children of an ever-changing life on the 'move'. Readers are able to follow the extraordinary career of the Australian Ian Howie, commencing in rural Bangladesh, followed by successive appointments to Sri Lanka, Kenya, Ghana, Rwanda, China, North Korea, Mongolia, Vietnam and the UN Headquarters in New York. Each chapter narrates the author's experience, in unvarnished prose, of living and working in each of these countries.

The book not only records achievements but also illustrates with examples where the UN has fallen short in the achievement of its development objectives. It isn't afraid to discuss failures and challenges from the past; in this, and many other ways, Ian Howie's memoirs perfectly bookends what has been achieved and how far there is yet to go. For the United Nations Population Fund (UNFPA), the author's primary employer, the book strategically prioritises the changes the author undertook throughout his various postings as he sought to move the Fund to fulfilling its mandate. It does so as UNFPA celebrated its 50-year anniversary since its founding, and the 25-year anniversary since the landmark International Conference on Population and Development (ICPD), which chartered the narrative around an individual's freedom to decide about their reproductive life, particularly for women, girls and young people.

Ian Howie's memoirs perfectly bookends what has been achieved and how far there is yet to go.

Joseph M. Siracusa
President Emeritus of Australia's Council for the Humanities Arts
and Social Sciences
Melbourne, Australia

Acknowledgements For someone with a history of finding transitions challenging I could never have managed the relocations demanded by a UN career without the love and support of my wife Alison. So often it falls to the "accompanying spouse" to establish a home base and find schools for the children. Alison achieved these and many other transitional challenges each time our family moved from one country to another.

My heartfelt thanks goes as well to those assisting me in digesting the content of my primary material plus helping me to research the countries covered, and the United Nations system. Included were student interns from RMIT University and the Australian Institute of International Affairs Victoria Division. I refer particularly to Ishita Acharyva, Madelaine Barry, Matilda Byrne, Lauren Fanning, Zoe Gelman–Malan, Maudie Farnan, Zachary Fletcher, Demian Freeman, Patrick Lamb, Catherine McLeod, Matilda Roeff, and Joseph Turnbull.

Also from RMIT university I would especially like to thank Professor Joe Siracusa, an internationally recognised author who never wavered in his support for my writing efforts including, once the manuscript was complete, applying his entrepreneurial flare to finding a publisher. Other RMIT colleagues such as Paul Battersby, Aya Ono and Aiden Warren were always helpful when it came to agreeing to intern support; and Sufia Begum assisted with the Bengali translations.

Past and current UN staff who provided valuable advice included: Bruce Campbell; Doreen Cross; Ian Davies; Cheikh Fall; Do Thi Thu Ha; Michael Henry; Yanming Lin; Gary Mcgillicuddy; Judy Phuong and Lynette Phuong. Their recollections added depth to my story.

Likewise my thanks for agreeing to be interviewed go to Peter Annear, Professor, Nossal Institute for Global Health, University of Melbourne; Erika Feller, Vice Chancellor's Fellow at The University of Melbourne and former Assistant High Commissioner (Protection), United Nations High Commissioner for Refugees (UNHCR); Gavin Jones, Emeritus Professor at the Australian National University; and Peter McDonald, Professor of Demography, University of Melbourne.

My appreciation goes as well to Annelies Kersbergen, Publishing Editor at Springer, Science+Business Media for accepting the manuscript and providing critical and strategic advice.

For professional advice I am indebted to Elisabeth Kerdelhué, Partnerships Manager, State Library Victoria; Margaret Sams Knight, business mentor; Cynthia Lloyd formerly with the Population Council; Debbie McInnes, public relations extraordinaire who, as a favour, went out of her way to link me in with potential publishers; Belinda Nemec, editor; Margie Seale, founder of the literary travel company Ponder & See; and Chris Shorten, Project Editor, Wiley Australia. I must also thank Gerald Caplan, public policy analyst and commentator for providing valuable country background advice and material.

For technical support I was often saved by Dawn Selkirk and Jason Sing. I also received constructive criticism from good friends John Box and Nick Green.

And, finally, I would like to thank my parents, Bruce and Mena, my brothers John and Ross, and their wives Linsey and Janet, who cared for my parents during my long absence.

Contents

Acronyms and Abbreviations

ACTs	Action Coordination Teams
AIDS	Acquired Immune Deficiency Syndrome
APRO	UNFPA's Asia Pacific Regional Office
ASRH	Adolescent Sexual and Reproductive Health
BARD	Bangladesh Academy for Rural Development
BCC	Behaviour Change Communication
CBD	Community-Based Distribution
CHG	Change Support Group
CICETE	China International Centre for Economic and Technical Exchanges
CO	Country Office
CP	Country Programme
CPAP	Country Programme Action Plan
CPR	Contraceptive Prevalence Rate
CSM	Contraceptive Social Marketing
CST	Country Support Team
CYP	Couple Years of Protection
DaO	Delivering as One
DHS	Demographic and Health Survey
EU	European Union
FAO	Food and Agriculture Organisation of the United Nations
FLE	Family Life Education
FP	Family Planning
GBV	Gender-Based Violence
GOV	Government of Viet Nam
GSO	General Statistics Office

HACT	Harmonised Approach to Cash Transfers
HIS	Health Information Systems
HIV	Human Immunodeficiency Virus
HOA	Heads of Agencies
HPPMG	Harmonised Programme and Project Management Guidelines
ICPD	International Conference on Population and Development
IEC	Information, Education and Communication
IFAD	International Fund for Agricultural Development
ILO	International Labour Organization
INGOs	International Non-Governmental Organizations
IOM	International Organisation for Migration
IPPF	International Planned Parenthood Federation
IUDs	Interuterine Devices
JPO	Junior Programme Officer
M&E	Monitoring and Evaluation
MCH	Maternal and Child Health
MDG	Millennium Development Goals
MIS	Management Information System
MOE	Ministry of Education
MOF	Ministry of Finance
MOFA	Ministry of Foreign Affairs
MOFTEC	Chinese Ministry of Foreign Trade and Economic Cooperation
MOH	Ministry of Health
MOHA	Ministry of Home Affairs
MOLISA	Viet Nam's Ministry of Labour, Invalids and Social Affairs
MPCFP	Bangladesh's Ministry of Population Control and Family Planning
MPI	Ministry of Planning and Investment
MPS	Ministry of Public Security
MSI	Marie Stopes International
MTR	Mid-Term Review
NCPFC	National Council on Population, Family, and Children
NGO	Non-Governmental Organisation
NPPP	National Project Professional Personnel
ODA	Official Development Assistance
OPF	One Plan Fund
PATH	Programme for Appropriate Technology in Health
PDS	Population and Development Strategies (UNFPA sub-programme)
PMT	Programme Management Team
PSI	Population Services International
RBM	Results-Based Management
RC	Resident Coordinator
RH	Reproductive Health
RHCS	Reproductive Health Commodity Security
RHIYA	Reproductive Health Initiative for Youth in Asia (EC-UNFPA initiative)

RTIS	Reproductive Tract Infections
SDG	Sustainable Development Goals
SMI	Safe Motherhood Initiative
SFPC	State Family Planning Commission
SRB	Sex Ratio at Birth
SRH	Sexual and Reproductive Health
STD	Sexually Transmitted Disease
TFR	Total Fertility Rate
TNTF	Tripartite National Task Force
TOT	Training of Trainers
UN	United Nations
UN Women	United Nations Entity for Gender Equality and the Empowerment of Women
UNAIDS	Joint UN Programme on HIV and AIDS
UNCT	United Nations Country Team
UNDAF	United Nations Development Assistance Framework
UNDG	United Nations Development Group
UNDP	United Nations Development Programme
UNEP	United Nations Environment Programme
UNESCO	United Nations Educational, Scientific and Cultural Organization
UNFPA	United Nations Population Fund
UN-Habitat	United Nations Human Settlements Programme
UNICEF	United Nations Children's Fund
UNIDO	United Nations Industrial Development Organization
UNODC	United Nations Office on Drugs and Crime
UNV	United Nations Volunteers
UNRC	United Nations Resident Coordinator
VCPFC	Viet Nam Commission for Population, Family, and Children
VINAFPA	The Viet Nam Family Planning Association
WB	World Bank
WFP	World Food Programme
WHO	World Health Organization
WFPE	Workforce Planning Exercise

1

From Melbourne and Back Again

More important is what you say when you finish rather than what you say when you start. Why? Because the past just does not disappear. It is evident everywhere.[1]

I feel uncomfortable when attention is focused on me. Moreover, conventional markers such as birthdays are nothing more than that. Markers. I simply see them as chronological goalposts measuring time passed but not those consequential events that may have happened on only one day or over the course of a number of years. Historical episodes may be time bound, but for those who are directly engaged they may never end.

Then again, when it comes to the United Nations' stand on population and development, it was 52 years in 2021 since the 1969 founding of my long-term employer, the United Nations Population Fund still known by its old acronym, UNFPA.[2] It was also 27 years since the Fund's landmark event, the International Conference on Population and Development (ICPD) was held in Cairo in 1994. These are significant historical markers. Their ramifications extend far beyond the actual events because both are lauded with consequences which continue to this day. For example, the ICPD's Programme of Action is commonly thought to have created a paradigm shift in how the global community regards population dynamics, moving from a focus on human numbers to a focus on human rights. Its agenda, particularly

---

[1] Unknown.
[2] United Nations Fund for Population Activities (UNFPA).

© The Author(s), under exclusive license to Springer Nature
Switzerland AG 2021
I. Howie, *Reflections on a United Nations' Career*, Springer Biographies,
https://doi.org/10.1007/978-3-030-77063-1_1

1

for women, girls, and young people, charted the path towards a new narrative based on an individual's freedom to decide about their reproductive life,

But when I returned to my hometown of Melbourne Australia in 2009, after an absence of 40 years, I found that most people had never heard of UNFPA let alone ICPD. Even within the development community, these acronyms produced interested but puzzled looks. UNFPA and ICPD may have been part of my everyday language, mantras rolling off the tongue, but what relevance did they have in a prosperous country not dependent on foreign aid? Even to those attuned to the UN, the organisation's many parts remained opaque. Still, people wanted to know what it was like to work for the UN. Students asked.[3] Audiences questioned. Family enquired. How did I start? Why did I choose it? What did I actually do? Did I make any difference? What was my favourite country? Would I recommend joining the UN? People were interested. They were thinking of a career or they wanted to know about the substance, the reality, and not the "pedantic gibberish of UN speak," as one colleague called it. Consequently, despite my reticence, I decided to write a book about the countries I had worked in, their circumstances at the time of my appointments, what I tried to do, and how well or otherwise I did it. I will tell how it started and what happened thereafter.

This book is a reflection. My aim is to create the truth of a thing (how it felt in me, my human experience), not the truth itself. My experiences were neither unique nor exceptional. Nearly all my UN colleagues, that is, those field-based ones, worked in a variety of countries and dealt with many challenges. That said, because of the UNFPA anniversaries, I feel a responsibility to set down what I learnt about the capacity of UNFPA the organisation to deliver on its mandate, and to do so at a time of celebration and a new reform agenda.[4] The reality was that the staff were not all a cluster of cutting-edge pioneers imbued with a commitment to the greater good of humanity, and the charisma and resources to step boldly forward. Rather, we were part of a UN bureaucracy which was, just that, a bureaucracy composed of civil

---

[3]Students marvel at my career seeing it as extraordinary which is something I never did. With their own futures in mind they want to know how I joined and what I did. They want to know what it was actually like.

[4]Initiated in 2017 by the UNFPA Executive Director, Natalia Kanem of Panama, who was appointed by the UN Secretary-General António Guterres on 3 October 2017. This followed consultations with the Executive Board of UNFPA which is made up of representatives from 36 countries elected on a regional basis—Africa, Asia and the Pacific, Eastern Europe, Latin America and the Caribbean and Western Europe and others.

servants drawn from all round the world, driven by a multiplicity of ambitions not all of which were related to the noblest of intentions.[5] Of course, the language we used (and still use) spoke in terms of saving people's lives and of tackling the great humanitarian challenges. And that, for a multilateral organisation, was right and proper. The UN is not a bilateral organisation advancing the causes of a particular state; it is the United Nations, a multilateral body consisting of agencies, funds and programmes whose mandates are rooted in the betterment of humankind. But having proclaimed these noble sentiments, those bureaucrats charged with delivering them are still, basically, bureaucrats—mostly good, well-intentioned individuals who struggle with an IN and OUT tray. Perhaps, in this regard, they are no different from any other staff members of a large global organisation. But, they need to be, for this is the UN and not a profit-driven multinational. As international civil servants we speak a universal mantra of human advancement, although as individuals our motivations for joining the organisation vary widely, as does our commitment to a global endeavour encompassing 193 countries. In the following chapters I try to separate the reality from the rhetoric and describe how it was.[6]

Looking back over my UN years, I wonder if I ever did anything meaningful or was I just another doomed dreamer. One, who, along with my colleagues, was instrumental in a self-deception, a bureaucratic operation essentially about nothing (other than our allowances). As I contemplate this, I feel a sense of disappointment that I never stood up or argued for a clearer

---

[5]From my experience, these may include access to a US green card, education of children in a privileged setting, a salary package well beyond that which was locally available and a well-endowed pension on retirement.

[6]In 2000, the Association of Former International Civil Servants (AAFI-AFICS) published a report: *What Happens to the Second Generation?* It endeavoured to define the community of international officials in the following manner. We live, generally, outside our own country. We are separated from our extended family and the society we were born into. We often work in a language that is not our own and is different from the language used in our own country. Our social life is with people from different countries, languages, societies, cultures, habits. We often end up marrying someone of a different nationality and culture; sometimes a marriage that would have lasted happily ever after in the home country, founders in alien climes. We may move about during our career and live in different countries. When we retire, we have to make a conscious choice of where to settle. And we might add to this list: We often feel more at home with our colleagues than with our compatriots. Yes, we are all this but aren't we something more as well? We have been moulded to a way of thinking, we see the problems of an increasingly interdependent world in a different manner, our viewpoint is no longer that of a particular nationality or tribe, we march to the beat of a different drum. Should we consider ourselves as rootless, cut off from the sap that nurtured us? Or should we consider ourselves as people who have accepted the planet as our homeland and discover that we are at home everywhere? In time, we may learn to look at the Earth as Neil Armstrong must have done on 21 July 1969 when he stepped on the Moon and took one giant step for mankind. We would see the oceans and the seas, the lakes and the rivers, the mountains and the glaciers, the deserts, and the forests—but we would not see the frontiers and the boundaries that divide nations and peoples. A career as an international civil servant would seem an ideal way to see global problems in a global context; the concept of an 'International Community' would become a living reality.

development line, one that I had tried and tested; that I never had the confidence to challenge bureaucratic policies and procedures which negated the UN's commitment to the poor. There were times when I didn't make the thoughtful calculations needed for tough decisions. Writing now, in part, absolves me for these failures, from a sense of shame.

Contributing to the urgency of documenting my working life is another reality. People are often ignorant of what happened five years ago, or when it comes to 'technical assistance'[7] what has been initiated in a neighbouring district or is about to be in another country. I recall reading with astonishment the thoughts of a British magistrate writing in the late 19th century about how best to support village development in rural Bangladesh. He knew from trial and error experience that a centralised location for accessing services, today's "one-stop shop", was a workable solution benefiting villagers.[8] But there is much repetition in development work, and it is a failure to not address the weaknesses of earlier efforts and build on the strengths. Ignorance should be no excuse for not knowing what is happening around you or what happened in the past. There is a literature which needs to be read. Development work should follow an upwards trajectory of improved delivery and not simply repeat all that has gone before, over and over again.

My UN experience began in 1976 with my appointment to the International Labour Organisation but, as one would expect, there was a prelude. Coming from a prosperous country like Australia I didn't just opt to go off on a whim to work among the rural poor in Bangladesh. The first conscious departure from the norm came earlier. It began with my entry into the competition for an American Field Service (AFS) scholarship to the United States.[9] My family was more surprised than I when I was successful and, for a family who had never travelled outside Australia, my departure in August 1963 for Fort Worth, Texas, was an emotional cleaver. The year I spent living with a host family and attending the local high school, in the company of my "American brother", was a transformative one. At age 17 how could it be otherwise? I was like a sponge absorbing newness every day. I was fully engaged as you would expect when catapulted away from the familiar routine

---

[7]A UN euphemism for aid via the use of technical advisers to a particular country.

[8]Better still, I thought, if we located that "shop" within the village and not at some distant location, thereby making it accessible and affordable.

[9]AFS Intercultural Programmes (or AFS, originally the American Field Service) is an international youth exchange organisation. It consists of over 50 independent, not-for-profit organisations, each with its own network of volunteers, professionally staffed offices, volunteer board of directors and website. In 2015, 12,578 students travelled abroad on an AFS cultural exchange programmes, between 99 countries. The U.S.-based partner, AFS-USA, sends more than 1,100 U.S. students abroad and places international students with more than 2,300 U.S. families each year. More than 424,000 people have gone abroad with AFS and over 100,000 former AFS students live in the U.S.

of a suburban life in Melbourne to a totally new environment where I had no past. I was no more the person who presented himself on day one. I was also the first exchange student my school had ever had. I was the exotic creature from faraway Australia.

Then there the multiple public speaking engagements during that AFS year in which I would talk of the importance of 'walking together, talking together, then and only then would we have world peace" (i.e., the AFS motto). I meant it. The other exchange students who joined me from Arlington and Dallas were proof of that relationship. They were from West Germany, Egypt and Argentina. We were mates. How could it be otherwise?

I had the first of my two encounters with history on the 22nd of November 1963. As an exchange student I was completing my final year at a high school in Fort Worth, Texas. The invitation to attend the breakfast given in honour of President Kennedy was arranged by a local congressman and rising Democratic star, Jim Wright.[10] The venue was the Crystal Ballroom of the Hotel Texas in downtown. We were asked to arrive early. Because it was cold and wet, I was there very early.[11] Fortunately, when seated, I was located close to the official table. I had easy viewing of all those who would be linked to that tragic affair—the President and the First Lady, Vice-President Johnson, and his wife "Lady Bird", and Governor Connally and Mrs Connally. Even now, fifty-seven years later, I can still see President Kennedy, Vice-President Johnson and Senator Yarborough entering via the hotel kitchen, just behind the official table (they did so for security reasons) to be followed some 25 min later by Mrs Kennedy. She was dressed in the same double-breasted, pink suit with blue trim and matching pink pillbox hat that became so famous. I described it all in a letter to my parents, writing of Jackie sitting there knowing that everyone was fixated on her. The President knew this too. When he opened his speech, he referred to himself as the man who accompanied Mrs Kennedy, adding that no-one ever paid any attention to what he wore. He then focused on defence and the role Fort Worth played in the US' military history.[12] For a president who was unpopular in the South West, this was smart politics or so I thought as an interested teenager. He was mending political fences. At the end of breakfast, it had been proposed that I would

[10]After serving as Majority Leader, Jim Wright became the 48th Speaker of the House, 1987–1989.

[11]Had I known that the President would greet crowds in the car park across the street from the hotel, I would have been even earlier.

[12]Carswell Field was a major Strategic Air Command (SAC) base during the Cold War. It was and is still located west of the central business district of Fort Worth. The Fort Worth Division of the General Dynamics Corporation (GD), an American aerospace and defence multinational corporation, was also critically important to the city.

be briefly introduced to the president, but such was the press of people that the prospect of the greeting had to be abandoned. The official party left by the same kitchen door. It was back at school when describing the event to my class that news filtered in of a shooting in Dallas. We were all in shock, trying to make sense of it all.

Later, Jim Wright, who had made that rendezvous with history possible, chaperoned me in Washington where we talked of how to make the world a better place (at least he did, and I again made precocious interventions). Later still, as part of the bus trip that brought all the exchange students under the AFS programme to both New York and Washington,[13] I recalled visiting the iconic UN Headquarters in midtown Manhattan. I was in the company of a West Indian doctor, his Jewish American wife, and their children. They were hosting me, the Australian exchange student who had spent his year in Texas. As I stood outside, looking up at the building on the East River, I thought maybe there was a future there. That experience sparked in me the possibility that the "walking and talking together," ideal espoused in the AFS motto, was not only a worthwhile personal goal but could also find expression in a career aimed at making a contribution.

When I returned home in 1964, reunited with my school friends in the final term of our school year, I knew I had changed. Inwardly I had but outwardly I was still the same tall skinny looking teenager now about to enter university. It was a period of confusion and alienation. I would try to artic- ulate a life spent 'over there' but after five minutes the conversation would inevitably turn to more local events. I was both different and still the same (not dissimilar to how I felt when I retired from the UN and returned to Melbourne after an absence of forty years). No doubt I came across as big- headed, not helped by the slow Texan drawl I had picked up. Those years were also a time of intense student agitation. By now I was a committed internationalist arguing against prejudice, racism, and militarism in all its forms. Underpinning this commitment were the philosophical writings of J. Krishnamurti, the Indian theosophist, with whom I closely identified. I also actively supported the Quaker position against the use of war as a means of solving international disputes. The outward manifestations of these beliefs were the stands I took against the white South African rugby tours, French nuclear tests in the South Pacific and the escalating wars in Laos and Viet Nam. I was a demonstrator. Then, when conscription for military service was

---

[13]While in Washington at an exchange student rally I directed a question to Attorney General Bobby Kennedy. I asked him about Jimmy Hoffa, the notorious Teamster leader, and what were his intentions.

introduced for all eighteen-year old's, I registered as a conscientious objector not knowing if I would be 'called up' or not. When my date of birth was one of those identified as requiring all young men born on that day to present themselves for military training, I refused. Following deferments to complete studies, I was finally summoned to appear in court and explain my actions. Not expecting to be granted an exemption, there being no precedent unless you could prove a religious objection, I argued my case on moral grounds, those espoused by the ambulance drivers who founded AFS and by the Quakers. I was adamant I would not serve and prepared myself to face the consequences (to the extent I understood what these would be). To my surprise, the magistrate granted me an exemption.

After graduation from Melbourne and Sydney universities with majors in economics and international relations I had to decide between progressing to a Ph.D. or applying for jobs which would see me working somewhere in the field of development. I chose the latter. I believed if I were to understand development, to get near the truth, I needed to work in a developing country. I made many job applications, covering many possibilities, with no luck. But, finally, I was successful. I went as a volunteer teacher to Fiji. My international career was under way. Later, I joined the Fiji Trades Union Congress as a volunteer Research Officer. It was an exciting time marked by a national strike over a trades dispute bill of the government which proposed a wage freeze along with legislation to curb industrial action. My lucky break with the UN came four years later. By now I was in Papua New Guinea working as an officer in the Department of Labour, Commerce, and Industry. It was 1976 and I was living in Port Moresby with my wife and her niece.

One day in Port Moresby I delivered a speech on behalf of my minister at the opening ceremony of an international conference. In the audience was a Bangkok representative of the ILO, one of the specialised agencies of the United Nations. After I finished speaking and the meeting adjourned for morning tea, the representative approached, and asked if I would be interested in going to work on a village-based project in rural Bangladesh. It was a pilot project, he said, aimed at translating agricultural progress into social transformation, principally through "Family Life Education (FLE)". "Truth be known, we are having trouble getting someone to go to rural Bangladesh especially now that that country had just had the worst outbreak of cholera in its history." He explained that being Australian was not relevant but that I spoke English and had a masters were. That I had never been to Bangladesh, knew virtually nothing about the country nor had any substantive expertise in the required subject area didn't seem to matter.

The ILO representative didn't need to ask me twice. I leapt at the opportunity. It didn't matter about the disease. It didn't matter about the potential isolation or the pending confrontation with poverty, corruption, and social dislocation. It also didn't matter that it was a contract, renewable annually for three years, and subject to the ongoing availability of finance and satisfactory performance. Nor did it matter that there was no guaranteed future once the contract ended and they flew me back to Melbourne. Working for the ILO under the umbrella of the UN was a dream come true (not that I knew they were connected at the time). I was idealistic if naïve. I was keen and willing to go. So it was that my UN career began.

During the next thirty years I was assigned to seven countries: Bangladesh, Sri Lanka, Kenya, Ghana, Viet Nam, China with responsibilities also for Mongolia and North Korea, and New York. I also undertook multiple short-term missions to many more countries and, since retirement, have undertaken special assignments for the UN in Rwanda and Papua New Guinea. Timing, career investment and promotion had much to do with where I was assigned. Each post had, and still has, a set duration according to the level of hardship. For example, Monrovia in Liberia is clearly different from Geneva in Switzerland.

While my years as a UN official may seem exotic to many, within the 'system' itself I did not see myself as any different from any of my colleagues. Sure, I came from a prosperous country, and had the luxury of middle-class idealism, and while others within the UN system were not as privileged as I, this was to be expected in an extended family of 193 nations. Besides, we could always go home to Australia.

My second rendezvous with a global tipping-point came thirty-eight years later to those tragic events in Dallas. After years assigned to developing countries, I found myself working and living in New York on 9/11, 2001. By a quirk of fate, it fell to me, as Chief of Human Resources for UNFPA, to evacuate our staff from their offices in the Daily News Building on the corner of 42nd Street and Second Avenue. On that day, my staff and I were scheduled to make a presentation of our biennial budget in the UN building on First Avenue. We were appearing before the UN's "Advisory Committee on Administrative and Budgetary Questions" (ACABQ).[14] We had arrived early. Being fully occupied, preparing, we were only vaguely aware of radio

---

[14]The Advisory Committee is an expert Committee of sixteen Members elected by the General Assembly for a period of three years, on the basis of a broad geographical representation. Members serve in a personal capacity and not as representatives of Member States. The Committee holds three sessions a year with total meeting time between nine and ten months per year. The programme of work of the Advisory Committee is determined by the requirements of the General Assembly and other legislative bodies to whom it reports.

reports that a plane had struck the twin towers on lower Manhattan. When a colleague's music was interrupted by a more urgent announcement, my immediate concern was that the UN building could be targeted. I telephoned UN security seeking advice about what was going on plus instructions on what we might need to do. They didn't reply! With no answer, I rushed back to our building on 42nd. As I entered our floor people looked to me as head of HR, presuming, I would know what to do. That wouldn't be the first time. But along with everybody else, I didn't know what was happening. Would there be more attacks and, if so, what would be targeted? I considered how the UN Building on the East River stood alone and exposed and how ours, the UNFPA offices one block away, could be also targeted if the goal was high-profile institutions. Then came the news that all transport to and from the island of Manhattan had been cut. The buses, ferries, subways, bridges, tunnels were closed. Time was pressing. I needed to take charge if we were going to evacuate our staff. What to do? I recalled that we had in every branch a staff member designated as the contact point for all other staff on any matters of Fund-wide significance. I contacted them with the instruction to link those who lived in Manhattan with two other colleagues who live in the boroughs.[15] Once the matching was made, we then evacuated down 23 flights of stairs. Outside we gathered at an agreed assembly point where I informed staff they couldn't go back to the building, but now needed to walk in threes to the homes of the Manhattan-based staff. They all began what was for many a very long walk. With the staff gone, the UNFPA Executive Director and I returned to her office and spent the rest of the day following events on television, wondering if the UN building would be the next target.[16] It was evening when I walked home along what were, by now, empty streets.[17] It was another decisive moment in modern American history.

---

[15]Later, UN staff from President Bush's designated "axis of evil" countries, North Korea, Iraq, Iran, Syria, Cuba and Libya would require special US government permission if they sought to travel beyond the five boroughs of New York.

[16]We never did hear from the "famed" UN blue helmets.

[17]A year later I had to again evacuate the building when it was presumed we were under threat. The Asia and Pacific Division had arranged a New York training programme among whose participants was a colleague from the Dhaka office in Bangladesh. When he arrived on the morning the training was to begin, his airline failed to locate his luggage. They sought advice from him as to where he would like his suitcase delivered when it arrived on the next flight. Not yet having booked a hotel, he gave the address of the UNFPA office, c/o the Daily News Building, 220 East 42nd Street between Second and Third. Later that day a van belonging to a courier service pulled up outside the building, parked illegally and the driver ran inside and dumped the suitcase. The people in reception looked at the labelling and then checked with our HQs staff listing but found no one of that name. "Isn't Muhammad Khan (not his actual name) a Muslim name?" said one receptionist to another. "I don't know but that suitcase looks suspicious. Evacuate the building and call the bomb-squad!" Once more I instructed staff to walk down the stairs and meet at the designated rallying point. Our Bangladeshi colleague trooped down along with everybody else oblivious that it was his suitcase

For me, as for most, these two historical snapshots have a significance more than the rare encounters they were. As a diplomat moving from country to country and mixing with the privileged élite, you are sometimes witness to major events and have the opportunity to meet with the national leadership. Whilst true in my case, these American-based happenings not only book-ended my career, they also marked significant points along it. They provided a context. They were markers before and after the nine countries I lived in; part of giving substance to a working life; an explanation for its twists and turns. I need to declare what I learnt from these and, more importantly, what they tell me of the capacity of the UN to deliver. When it came to be writing this memoir, I did not want to write as a cynic, to reveal warts and all of what I knew of the UN system. I didn't want to malign my colleagues nor denigrate the organisation. I'm loyal. The UN is a body worth fighting for. It can do extraordinary things. But in my view, it can do better, and it should be doing better. Because its mission has stalled—witness the declining financial base with the rise of other development players—I feel I have a responsibility to tell my experiences where it relates, albeit in a small way, to reforming the organisation. Perhaps, as I write, some sort of understanding may emerge, something meaningful on which the UN can build. So, this book is something I feel compelled to do, to record my journey, my self-education, because I owe it to the UN as an organisation I believe in and am committed to. It is essential in the management of globalisation.

The book is organised according to most of the countries in which I served. Not all. I have excluded some where my experience added little to the mandate of UNFPA. Additionally, when I look at my UN career I think in terms of countries, rather than the actual years I was in each of them. I have found that when I have to recall specific dates and times I have to pause and do a mental calculation. But mention a country and it evokes recollections of individuals met and experiences lived irrespective of the year and actual duration. It is more than the geographic name. That is only a title on a map. It is what it means that I want to recall.

---

about to be examined by the bomb-squad. Outside I again instructed everybody to go home, leaving any personal effects at their desk. Fortunately, the suitcase didn't explode, and it was collected the following day.

I follow those postings where I have been challenged in my efforts to make a difference and, in doing so, I talk of my personal experiences against the background of the country as it was at the time of my appointment. Given the varied intensity of these experiences, my chapters fluctuate in length. They also reveal how, over time, my knowledge of how the UN functioned along with insights into how it could function, changed as my role changed.

My obsession with taking notes and recording meetings and discussions provides the major source for the content. Taking notes can upset people but I was always careful when it was a one-on-one meeting to seek their permission before I produced my notebook.[18] But, like any other jottings, these notes are not always accurate recordings or verbatim shorthand. Some are just observations and reflections as they occurred to me at the time or were taken with the advantage of hindsight. Moreover, my ability to record also changed over time. Supporting the earlier chapters are the letters written to my parents. Later observations came in the emails I wrote to my wife without whom I could not have pursued my UN career and to whom I have an everlasting debt of gratitude.

The account begins with my appointment to the ILO in 1976. It ends in 2012 with the last of my UN assignments. It flows chronologically as I navigate from one country to another. It also moves from my position of virtual ignorance of the organisation I was so keen to join, to an increased understanding of its multiple layers plus insights into its cast of characters. Of course, there are generalisations made which may be uncomfortable for some and questionable by others. It is, after all, a personal narrative but also a contribution. A contribution to what? Development? Global understanding? The poor? A liberal political agenda? As a UN staff member over a period of more than thirty years, I was charged with delivering programmes of development, ones directed, specifically towards poor marginalised women. It may be a digital world now, but I want to look at things as I saw them and not what the press releases, the web sites, say they were. Did I succeed? Did we succeed? By reflecting on my assignments in this book, I want to know the answer. Of course, I make no claim to being unbiased or always accurate. I offer vignettes. Random thoughts, observations and insights inevitably mean a skewed, disparate, eccentric, and one-dimensional

---

[18]Where possible I have deliberately avoided naming names. Not surprisingly having spent so many years in the system including being in charge of personnel for 7 years, I know a lot about a lot of people. But I have no wish to air dirty linen, to tittle-tattle, to gossip and besmirch individuals. Besides, it would be only my view and I may be wrong. More to the point this book is about the UN system as a collective of agencies, funds and programmes of which the staffing profile, its characteristics and the milieu in which they work is more important than the individuals who make it up.

record. Beginning as they do in the 1970s, they may seem quaint to a contemporary reader. But I suspect that little has changed in the way the UN conducts its development business. And, therein lies the challenge, and part of the reason I am writing this book. Given the paucity of autobiographical writing by my peers, scrutiny of the UN system may profit from the recollections of one retired staff member's experience and analysis.

2

Welcome to the UN Family

"For me, it was like plunging into another world, one where people spoke peculiar languages, in all of which they tossed around strange acronyms while bantering about meetings and reports from the past (and) United Nations subdivisions" **Katherine Graham**[1]

"Welcome to the UN family," the ILO representative said. When I looked puzzled, he added, "The ILO is a specialised agency of the United Nations." "Is it?" I replied. I knew the organisation was a tripartite body composed of employer, employee, and government representation. I also knew that Australian union stalwart and future Prime Minister, Bob Hawke and the well-known employers' advocate, George Polites, were regular attendees at the annual ILO conferences. I knew it was headquartered in Geneva, but part of that New York based UN system? That I didn't know.

In fact, there was an enormous amount I didn't know. Chief among these was the ability of my wife and niece to undertake the transition and cope with the dynamics of change. We were leaving extended families plus the familiarity of Australia and the South Pacific. It was a plunge into the unknown. Then, there was the task I was being assigned to where it was assumed I had the requisite technical knowledge, which I clearly didn't.[2] In the telexes now

---

[1] Katherine Graham, PERSONAL HISTORY (Vintage Books, New York), 1997, p. 587.

[2] An assumption I came to realise was common throughout the UN system but one which was generally unquestioned because it applied to so many or because it was assumed you were never going to find the perfect fit anyway, especially in a hardship post. Moreover, most of us adjusted our CVs to the advertised vacancy and hoped, if selected, we would learn it all on the job.

© The Author(s), under exclusive license to Springer Nature Switzerland AG 2021
I. Howie, *Reflections on a United Nations' Career*, Springer Biographies,
https://doi.org/10.1007/978-3-030-77063-1_2

being exchanged my new title read "Expert on Rural Development Cooperatives and Family Life Education"; Executing Agency—International Labour Organisation; Implementing Agency—Bangladesh Academy for Rural Development (BARD); Location—Comilla (i.e. eighty kilometres south east of the capital, Dhaka); Funding Agency—United Nations Fund for Population Activities (UNFPA). Those were a lot of partners I was answerable to. It suggested I knew a lot about Bangladesh, the country, and its history. I didn't, nor did I know a lot about cooperatives or family planning hidden as it was under that euphemism, "Family Life Education". I now needed to do some quick research. I rushed to the library. I also sought out people who had worked for the UN, been to Bangladesh or better still were Bangladeshi. There was not a lot available, although I did read about the impact the oil crisis was having on development and the establishment of the G7 to promote better coordination. There were also reports from the global conferences on the environment (Stockholm, 1972) and women (Mexico City, 1975). The club of Rome, established in 1974, seemed to have some relevance. Still, I was sure the members of the ILO Regional Labour and Population Team for Asia and the Pacific (LAPTAP), based in Bangkok, would be able to provide me with the expert knowledge required. More telexes followed, including one whereby my wife's niece, for whom I was the guardian, was now officially accepted as my dependent. When Thai Airways called to say that our travel authorisation had been received, Moresby/Bangkok/Geneva/Dhaka, we were ready to go. The adventure was under way.

For each of the Bangkok and Geneva ILO briefings it was assumed I would know where to stay and, once arrived, be able to navigate my way around the cities and the multiple UN offices. Unlike embassy postings, the ILO at that time didn't begin briefing appointees months in advance, nor did it arrange accommodation, unless asked, or attend to other personal matters. The practice was that you were assigned a date for departure, two or three days were allocated for briefings (at the regional office and HQ's) and then you started. Now that I was in Bangkok, it was expected that I would find my way to the ESCAP[3] building where the LAPTAP Team was located. Later, in Geneva at ILO HQ, I would repeat the same procedure. All perfectly reasonable or so it seemed at the time.

On Day One, suitably suited, I set out. The ESCAP building was a grand structure. Fronted by low conference rooms resplendent with flags from many countries, it rose up behind a multi-story office building. At the entrance I met my first blue helmet, those tight shirted UN security guards who protect,

---

[3]United Nations Economic and Social Commission for Asia and the Pacific.

or otherwise, UN premises and dress in the fashion of American policemen. I asked him where to go. Everyone else, streaming past, seemed to have the answer. They walked with commitment, authoritatively pressing lift buttons to their designated floors. I felt inadequate feeling that somehow the "knowledge" had passed me by. The guard gave me the appropriate directions. To my surprise, when I found the correct floor and nervously walked through the central open-planned area, looking to see if I could recognise a name posted on office doors, I was greeted by a diminutive Thai woman who handed me my schedule of appointments. She was a member of the local general staff as distinct from the international professional cadre and, as I was to discover, was pivotal to the running of that office. Lesson one—you can do without a boss, but you can't do without your personal assistant. My schedule showed there was a meeting with a different technical adviser, every hour on the hour. This was a challenging but impressive agenda for Day One. But later on, that first day, when I met the team leader, it wasn't in his office but in the VIP dining room of the building (preferred to the staff cafeteria), over a long lunch complete with alcohol. Gone was the schedule because all my appointees were there around the table. Over lunch I laughed along with everybody else at stories or jokes I sometimes struggled to understand. I was an outsider and not for the first time was ashamed of my mumbled acquiescence as I joined in. I found them to be an eclectic lot despite their uniform dress code of safari suits. There was a Sri Lankan Burgher from his national employers' association, an Indian who began his career in the ILO office New Delhi, a Welshman with an academic background in population, a Sikh gentleman from the Indian provincial bureaucracy and a South Korean who was known by his initials, his surname being incredibly common.[4] There were no women other than those serving in the general staff, where they were all women. Like me, the professionals had been recruited by ... actually, I didn't know. Was it by word of mouth, a chance connection, a personal reference, a friend's wink and a nod, or a vigorous application process? I never did find out but when compared to my uncertain first steps all my colleagues seemed totally confident. They knew the rituals like some secret society into which one had to be initiated.

The organisational structure was hierarchical with the leader holding the floor and each of us agreeing to his approach. I soon found out that the 'game', for that's what it was, wasn't that difficult once you accepted the parameters and learnt the language. For example, I assumed all my colleagues were experts in their discipline with years of field experience, an impressive list

---

[4] A number of these staff fluctuated between the ILO's Geneva and Bangkok offices.

of publications and senior positions held earlier in their respective countries. Surely, they had been headhunted to join the committed few charged with advancing the UN's development agenda. This turned out to be not quite true. What they were, were UN bureaucrats, skilled and efficient at playing the game, outwardly committed to the issues, replete with the language, able to navigate the corridors and comfortable in the knowledge they were going to be in the system for a long time. Like me, there were many who didn't know all that much about development theory nor the technical specialisation we were working in, namely, population education and family planning. We had all learnt it on the job or were about to in my case and gave lip service to sounding authoritative. But within the broader UN tent, LAPTAP was an efficient operation and not without its committed individuals. What I now needed to learn was why the ILO was about to "execute" a project funded by UNFPA in rural cooperatives in Bangladesh? Wasn't the ILO a tripartite body dedicated to advancing the cause of labour rights through international conventions and global resolutions?[5] Where a country struggled to meet these obligations, the ILO then provided the technical assistance to support their efforts in reaching the desired level enunciated in the given convention.

But who was UNFPA, the funding agency? Now known simply as the UN Population Fund, I read that when it became operational in 1969[6] it was known as the United Nations Fund for Population Activities, UNFPA. I knew there was a link to demography, essentially the study of population, from the useful and highly regarded demographic information published in the annual State of World Population report.[7] I was now to learn that UNFPA was the lead UN agency addressing the sexual and reproductive health needs of women and girls. I came to see the Fund as providing women with choices in their lives, including those related to reproduction and sexual health. In fact, the goal of the Fund was to change people's behaviour and to help individuals make their own decisions about the number and timing of the children they had. From my research I read that the initial calls for reproductive planning were thought to have originated in the mid-1940s, after the post-World War II population boom. It was around 1950 when sociologists

---

[5]International labour standards, which are made up of Conventions, Protocols to Conventions and Recommendations, are universal instruments agreed to by the international community and reflect common values and principles on work-related issues. While ILO member States can choose whether or not to rectify an ILO Convention, the ILO considers it important to keep track of developments in all countries, whether or not a state has ratified them.

[6]Earlier, in 1967, UN Secretary General U Thant proposed a fund that would assist in areas related to population, including research, training, and advising.

[7]2016s report focused on the 60 million girls aged 10 around the globe, and 2017's centred on the growing gap between the world's richest and poorest.

and biologists first grew concerned that the world was bursting at the seams with humans, to the detriment of the environment, and called for something to be done.[8] Adding fuel to these anxieties was the US government's fear that poor countries in Asia were fertile ground for communist revolutions.[9] It was the Lyndon Johnson administration, especially US Defence Secretary Robert McNamara, that articulated the most concern about growing populations. New macroeconomic models then persuaded government economic planners that rapid population growth posed a serious threat to raising per capita incomes.[10] Important to recall, however, that this was challenged by some economists, who claimed development was not hindered by rapid population growth.[11] Nonetheless, UNFPA was created in 1967 as a trust fund and at the 1968 International Conference on Human Rights, family planning became a human rights' obligation of every country, government and policymaker. The conference outcome document, known as the Tehran Proclamation, stated unequivocally: "Parents have a basic human right to determine freely and responsibly the number and spacing of their children"—Article 16. By 1969, it was unanimous. Unchecked population growth impeded development. The fear was real and in that same year the agency began operations as UNFPA under the administration of the United Nations Development Programme (UNDP). In 1971 it was placed under the authority of the UN General Assembly. It had now emerged from a tiny forum in the 1950s to a separate fund.

But its creation, even then, was not without controversy. Surprisingly, in light of later events, it was a Republican President, Richard Nixon, who maintained that the UN should take the lead on population issues,[12] and another Republican President, George H. W. Bush, then the US ambassador to the UN, who advocated strong support for the UN to launch a population

---

[8]This timing does not ignore the pioneer efforts by Margaret Sanger, Marie Stopes, and others in the early part of the Twentieth Century to provide birth control in the urban settings of the US and the slums of the UK.

[9]In 1959 the Draper Committee's report, commissioned to study the impacts of US military aid, suggested that the US should become involved in trying to slow population growth in developing countries. Rachel Sullivan Robertson "UNFPA in Context: An Institutional History" Background paper prepared for the Centre for Global Development Working Group on UNFPA's Leadership Transition, October 2010. pages 5–7.

[10]The view that population growth was a 'problem' was widely shared among many of the leading figures within UNDP, including Richard Symonds (who was hired by Sec-General U Thant to write a report on the UN's past and future population roles) and David Owen (who moved from UNDP to head the International Plan Parenthood Federation). Craig N. Murphy, THE UNITED NATIONS DEVELOPMENT PROGRAMME A BETTER WAY? (Cambridge University Press, Cambridge, 2006), pp 163–164.

[11]Keyfitz 1990.

[12]Betsy Hartmann, REPRODUCTIVE RIGHTS AND WRONGS: THE GLOBAL POLITICS OF POPULATION CONTROL (South End Press), 1995.

programme.[13] Still more Republicans, such as General William Draper, the US delegate to the UN Population Commission, 1969–71, were interested in a multilateral body to address population growth in developing countries. They wanted something practical, feeling the UN's Population Division was too technical and academic to carry out this role.[14] Knowing the controversy related to family planning and population issues they argued for a fund reliant on voluntary rather than mandatory contributions.

Within the UN system itself all was not supportive either. Fears of excessive bureaucracy and duplication led to questions whether a separate organisation was needed with the World Health Organization (WHO) arguing that family planning should be incorporated into their larger health efforts. Fifty years later, 2019, UNFPA's anniversary, little had changed.

When it came to who would be UNFPA's first executive director, the then Administrator of UNDP, Paul Hoffman, persuaded Rafael Salas, the executive secretary of President Ferdinand E. Marcos of the Philippines and a Roman Catholic, to join UNDP, New York, in 1968 as a population consultant. Based on his preliminary work on funding and staffing, Salas became the first Executive Director (ED) of UNFPA in 1969, a position he held until 1987. Although I never met Mr Salas, he is widely acknowledged to have put UNFPA on the map by focusing on the population element and given the fear of a population time bomb, raising the launching capital.

In 1987, Salas was followed by Nafis Sadik, a Pakistani doctor and UNFPA division director, who held the post of ED from 1987 to 2000. Dr. Sadik is credited with switching the focus of the Fund to reproductive health and sexuality, a more clinical approach. There were two distinct trains of thought prior to this that had permeated the population and development debate—individual choice versus societal needs. Pioneers of the birth control movement, such as the American Margaret Sanger, were largely concerned with the right of each woman to make decisions about her own body and her own fertility. This was a moral argument, rather than an economic one, and one that was reinforced by the UN. Those in the societal needs' camp were more concerned about the effect of rapid population growth on poverty, the availability and use of natural resources, and economies across the world. The thinking was that a stable population could share the rewards of economic growth better than any overpopulated place could. These two streams of global family planning, individual choice, or greater

---

[13]Peter J. Donaldson, NATURE AGAINST US: THE UNITED STATES AND THE WORLD POPULATION CRISIS, 1965–1980, 1990.

[14]Stanley Johnson, WORLD POPULATION AND THE UNITED NATIONS: Challenge and Response (Cambridge University Press, Cambridge) 1987.

collective benefit were at odds with one another. In 1974 at the third World Population Conference held in Bucharest, the focus was on the relationship between population size, economics and societal development.[15] The Conference adopted a World Population Plan of Action, which contained for the first time a recommendation stating that

> All couples and individuals have the right to decide freely and responsibly the number and spacing of their children and to have the information, education and means to do so; the responsibility of couples and individuals in the exercise of this right takes into account the needs of their living and future children, and their responsibilities towards the community.[16]

It was also in Bucharest that the Bangladesh representative made a passionate speech, outlining the problems his country faced as one of the world's most densely populated states. With a fertility rate of seven children per woman in 1972 with only 10% of married couples being provided with contraceptives, it was this plea which was said to have been instrumental in saving the meeting from breaking up in disarray.[17] Ten years later, the second International Conference on Population in Mexico City advanced the belief that rapidly developing technology would be able to meet and then overcome future limits to resources. The assumption was that humankind would overcome any challenge and the planet could accommodate vast numbers. Jump forward another ten years, to the International Conference on Population and Development in Cairo (ICPD) in 1994, 18 years after I joined the ILO, and the thinking had shifted to individual reproductive health. The focus was

---

[15]This Conference, the first of an intergovernmental nature, was attended by representatives of 135 countries. The Second World Population Conference was organized in 1965 by the International Union for the Scientific Study of Population (IUSSP) and the United Nations. It was held in Belgrade and most of the participants were experts in the field. The focus was on the analysis of fertility as part of a policy for development planning. This Conference was held at a time when expert studies on the population aspects of development coincided with the start-up of population programmes subsidized by the United States Agency for International Development (USAID). The First World Population Conference organised by the United Nations was held in Rome in 1954 to exchange scientific information on population variables, their determinants, and their consequences. As an academic conference it resolved to generate more information on the demographic situation of developing countries and to promote the creation of regional training centres which would help to address population issues and prepare specialists in demographic analysis. Source: ECLAC.

[16]World Population Plan of Action, August 1974, Adopted by the World Population Conference, Bucharest, 1974, Section B. Principles and objectives of the Plan, paragraph 14 (f).

[17]Stanley Johnson, THE POLITICS OF POPULATION: CAIRO 1994 (Earthscan Publications Ltd, London), 1995 pp. 75–76.

now on choice with the timing, spacing and number of children being a decision made between informed and consenting adults, and not one directed by governments.[18] That was the position advanced by Dr. Sadik.

While individual choice was to become the rhetoric post-Cairo, in 1976 when I joined the UN, both the ILO and UNFPA, being agents of the system, were required to support the implementation of government policies. In my case this meant working with two ministries. The Bangladesh Ministry of Health and Population Control, as it was then called but, given the reference to control, now no longer considered an appropriate title, and the Ministry of Local Government, Rural Development and Co-operatives. But what did these two ministries have in common? More to the point, how did population relate to cooperatives? If I were to work in this field, I needed to know.

Like many realities in the UN there was a perfectly plausible explanation: money.[19] Historically, the ILO had always viewed cooperatives as important. They were seen as a vehicle for improving the living and working conditions of women and men globally, as well as making essential infrastructure and services available even in areas neglected by the state and investor-driven enterprises. It was through this institutional base that the ILO saw one of their key goals of "technical cooperation" being achieved. But, as I was to discover, the ILO branch charged with this responsibility as it related to the cooperative movement was, despite the rhetoric, small and underfunded. When an opportunity presented itself to access UNFPA funds for an "Information, Education and Communication" (IEC) initiative through rural cooperatives that would advance "family life education" (FLE), the link was made via Geneva, Bangkok and Dhaka, and the funds advanced to the ILO as part of the UNFPA Programme of Assistance to the Government

---

[18]The third Executive Director of UNFPA and the second who I came to know personally was Thoraya Obaid. Thoraya, a Saudi national, was the first Saudi Arabian woman to receive a government scholarship to study at a university in the United States (she has a doctorate degree in English Literature and Cultural Anthropology). Prior to joining UNFPA, she was Deputy Executive Secretary with the United Nations Economic and Social Commission for Western Asia (ESCWA) where she had begun her career in 1975. It was from 1998 to 2001, when she was Director, Division for Arab States and Europe, that I first met Thoraya. Indeed, it was as Chief, Human Resources that I contacted Dr. Obaid to solicit her interest in joining UNFPA.

[19]Later, I read that when the first Executive Director of UNFPA, Rafael M. Salas, made his initial visit to the ILO he "...found the officials of this organisation very receptive to the idea of opening up new undertakings in population, particularly as ILO was passing through a period of acute financial stringency and the prospect of funded projects via population was especially attractive (p 38)...(the Organisation) started an exploration of vocational training and cooperative rural development programs to see how they could be adjusted to take in the new element (p. 45)". Rafael M. Salas, PEOPLE: AN INTERNATIONAL CHOICE The Multilateral Approach to Population (Pergamon Press, Oxford), 1977.

of Bangladesh. Whilst I can explain all this now, at the time it was all very confusing and it remained that way for a long time.[20]

What I also did not understand was that there was separation between the executing agency, the implementing agency, and the funding agency. What was this all about? Who was driving what? Was it the government, the agency, or the donor? Something else I didn't know nor was I sufficiently insightful then to see, were the contradictions and the overlaps. Perhaps the answer would come in Geneva. After a night out on the town in Bangkok with my new colleagues, I was off to ILO Headquarters. It was goodbye to LAPTAP, hello to EMP/POP ILO Geneva and welcome to the alphabet soup of the United Nations.

For my first visit, Geneva was something of a surprise. After Bangkok, the airport was quiet and low key and, to my surprise, the taxi driver wore a jacket and tie, and drove a Mercedes. The hotel, picked randomly because of its proximity to the central bus station, was, incongruously or so it seemed to me, named The Windsor. The bedroom was small, the lift groaned and the surrounding neighbourhood less than salubrious. It gave me a sense that I may have been repeating the arrival of a first-time visitor to the League of Nations pre-war. It all seemed very European, especially the continental breakfast served daily—fresh crisp rolls, butter, berry jam and slices of ham and cheese. After the meal on that first morning I headed out to catch the bus at the central station to the ILO office. But which bus and where to get on and off? I did not know, nor had the office provided any guidance for the uninitiated. I assumed they assumed I'd know. As in Bangkok, this didn't seem unreasonable. Everyone at the bus stop seemed to know where they were going except me. I followed the suits.

The ILO office in Geneva was a very grand angular building located in parkland. Completed in 1974, the building with its façade of glass and cast aluminium consisted of 6 floors, 1250 offices, more than 2,000 staff and very long corridors. Following my walk from the bus stop, endeavouring to appear earnest and propelled along with those who obviously were, I entered the lobby. Again, I had to rely on the blue helmet seated at the front entrance

---

[20]The UN is a complex organisation. Rather like a confederation it consists of autonomous intergovernmental organisations all linked to the Economic and Social Council (ECOSOC) which in turn reports to the General Assembly (GA). The specialised agencies were established by formal intergovernmental treaties the same way the UN was. A number predate the establishment of the UN such as the ILO which was founded in 1919. They are financed according to levies on their member states. The 'operational' agencies of the UN, such as UNDP, UNICEF, WFP and UNFPA are basically funded by voluntary contributions, mainly from governments. They were established by resolutions of the GA to extend aid to developing countries. Their executive heads, unlike those of the specialised agencies, are appointed by the Secretary-General of the UN. Agency heads are elected and are answerable to their own governing bodies.

on where to go. As I didn't speak French, it was a bit of a challenge, but I was learning to be self-reliant and to figure it out. I did not question what was, for me at least, a lack of ILO preparation, but later I asked myself whether it was incompetence, a lack of sensitivity or perhaps a working demarcation between the concerns of headquarters and those of the field. I didn't know but when I was told they could not find anyone prepared to go to rural Bangladesh it occurred to me there were two games at play: the ILO proposing population-related solutions to different governments and then, in order to attract the requisite funding, advocating for their inclusion in a country programme funded by UNFPA. Indeed, all the ILO regional and global population projects inclusive of the Bangkok and Geneva staff, were funded by UNFPA, and it was by this means that these long serving international civil servants maintained their positions. The country projects they initiated, once signed, and funded, were how they justified continuation. There was no doubt they were able to competently handle a file, even many in fact, but it was not development transforming the lives of the poor. It was administration in the name of humanitarian causes from the comfort of Geneva, New York, and Bangkok. It was a triumvirate among a coterie of individuals who used the language of behavioural change, thereby appealing to UN funding agencies and their potential country donors.[21] Not that I saw this at the time. Only later when based in New York did I see the near impossibility of relocating long-serving staff away from their settled life in the suburbs to the front lines of development. What I did see back in 1976 was that it was now up to me as to whether or not my pilot project achieved the goals set, located as I soon would be, in a rural corner of a developing country. Did I assume then that if I served my time, reported positively, and received glowing accounts from my counterparts and superiors, I, too, would advance to the funded security of a regional or headquarters' office? It didn't, although in retrospect it was not without its appeal—I would have welcomed an appointment to Geneva. But back then I still had a lot to learn.

What followed in Geneva during this initial briefing was a series of appointments, all with people who were new to me. They followed a pattern the content of which I would become very familiar with over the years. I would be issued with a typed sheet containing the names of officers to be meet, their designations, the time of the appointment and its location. Mostly my appointments were given over to people talking about what they

---

[21]That said, a balanced scorecard on the UN would need to record that many of the new concepts on development now being advocated had their origins in ILO thinking. Take, for example, the concept of basic needs which was introduced by the ILO in the seventies and under whose umbrella we were initiating our development efforts.

were doing at HQ. There were also those who I was required to meet in order to complete important paperwork. Would I be applying for an education grant for my niece? Where did I want my salary paid? What about the mandatory proportion that had to be paid in-country and in local currency? Where would that go? For the remainder, what would be my bank account in Geneva? It was suggested I think carefully about this because exchange rates varied over time as well as from the point of origin to the point of receipt. Really? I hadn't ever thought about any of these questions. I had mostly anticipated briefings on Bangladesh. But there was nothing handed over on the history of the country, its demographic profile and the population challenges faced. No country plans were copied. Nor was any literature forthcoming on the economy, culture, Islam and what other donors, including the UN, were doing. Did they assume I would gather this myself or that I knew it already? I didn't know but I suspected they didn't have it. It was not within their frame of reference. This was a headquarters' briefing not a field one. Whatever the case, I always seemed to be dashing along corridors, reading name plates over closed doors, and arriving late, usually out of breath. Lunch was equally an adventure. I somehow found my way to the staff cafeteria, that there was one was a novelty, and once there lined up with my tray pretending to be totally familiar with the procedure. Because everyone I enquired from was invariably polite and understanding I came to see that my rushed behaviour must have been the norm. For this the urbanity of the support staff particularly struck me. They seemed so sophisticated switching as they did from one language to another. There was a sense of history here, a quiet certitude with an established routine, even if I couldn't quite grasp it. Coming from wealthy Australia I also wondered how other new appointees from less privileged backgrounds managed their briefings. Were they as confused as I was, trying to figure who was who and where to go? Like me, I assumed they were all keen and just wanted to get on with the job.

After long days running down those endless corridors, searching for the right name on the right door, and after making multiple but muffled enquiries about what was going on, my day's appointments would come to an end. I would leave the headquarters and walk out of the building across the substantial lawns to the bus stop. There, I expected to see crowds of colleagues waiting for the bus and chatting away about important matters. But there was rarely anyone. Where did they all go? I heard that many lived in France where it was cheaper and drove to and from work. I also hoped, being a new appointee, that someone would have asked me for a drink in the evening or even a meal at home but there were no invites. But I didn't mind. I did resolve, however, that whenever a colleague visited me at my duty station, wherever that might be, I would always invite them home for dinner; a commitment I honoured throughout my international career. For my first time in Geneva though, I was simply in awe at being there and determined to see all I could.[22] Next stop, Dhaka, the antithesis of an orderly, affluent European city.

---

[22]On the weekends I walked and walked and became an expert at catching buses to distant places. For an Australian who basically only spoke English, the ability of the drivers to switch from French to German to Italian to English seemed remarkable. They mirrored the staff at the ILO. Later, while my language deficiencies were always an impediment and how I would have relished switching into another tongue (even my 'street speak' was always well received), working in ex British colonies made life easier. English was commonly spoken, there were connections such as cricket through a shared British heritage, the BBC was available 24/7 and the international community were just that, a community.

3

Learning by Doing: Bangladesh

"You can't cross the sea merely by standing and staring at the water".
Rabindranath Tagore

Our arrival in Dhaka was a shock. There were three of us, including myself, my then wife and my teenage niece. We were not mentally prepared for the heat, the dust, and the squalor. On arrival, the aggression of the customs' officials as they vetted our belongings primed our sense of unease. We were instantly suspicious of all around us. It didn't help that after being jostled inside the airport terminal, we were then confronted in the car park by what seemed to be a surging crowd fixated on us: rickshaw drivers all shouting to choose them in a cacophony of sound and waving of arms. This included a naked beggar who immediately approached us, arms outstretched, pleading and prostrating himself.[1] We instantly drew back only to be tapped on the leg by a child sheltering under a car.[2] She rubbed her stomach and then moved her hand to her mouth indicating that she was hungry and needed food. Survival was what it seemed to be all about. Later on, and by then partially immune to the poverty, we simply accepted it, and learnt how to respond to crowds of outstretched arms. "*Maaf Koren,*" we would say, "Please forgive us,

---

[1]Later, as I travelled in and out of the country, I came to know this man and I regularly saved a little something for him.

[2]Unlike today's congested streets there were not many cars on Dhaka's streets back in the seventies.

© The Author(s), under exclusive license to Springer Nature
Switzerland AG 2021
I. Howie, *Reflections on a United Nations' Career*, Springer Biographies,
https://doi.org/10.1007/978-3-030-77063-1_3

we cannot give," the standard Islamic response to a request for alms. Once heard, the beggars would quietly move on looking elsewhere for charity.

It was a chaotic introduction. Not only was there no-one to meet us but as we taxied away from the airport, crowds, noise, and poverty seemed to close in. When we stopped at traffic lights, men would tap against the windows of our car. It was a never-ending sea of unsmiling male faces, up close, openly staring, commenting, and pointing. We drew back but how to escape. In my early letters to my parents, I asked them to imagine a society where the poor learnt their survival skills as early as learning to walk. Most seemed to live by their wits in the struggle to survive. Add to this that half the population (i.e., the women) were physically removed from public life and that those you did see were purdah-clad, relegated to second place and culturally certain that boys could behave in a way their sisters would never be allowed to. Only later did you come to see the standard dress for women, the two-piece *shalwar kameez*,[3] as a colourful tradition. We saw it initially as an outfit intended to deny basic femininity. These were societal practices none of us had ever been exposed to. Like many foreigners before us, it would have been easy to draw in on ourselves and become resentful and condemnatory. We did not see a society steeped in Tagore, risen from a liberation war, struggling with the aftermath of famines, and adjusting to coups and countercoups.[4] There were just crowds of bigoted men seeking to condemn. Later, I would write of the fixated stare of an unworldly villager at seeing a foreign man and women walking together and the obsequious behaviour of others seeking to curry favour from the foreigner—the piques of jealousy and the looks of envy at what was seen as our better circumstances. It was at once instant and overwhelming—a dramatic confrontation with the resulting rush to judgement. We were simply unprepared for what was to become our life in this country. Our western frame of reference was being attacked and

---

[3]A long flowing tunic worn over the top of matching balloon style baggy pants and finished with an *orna* (a loose scarf) draped over a woman's chest.

[4]On November 12, 1970, a cyclone hit Bangladesh leading to the death of an estimated 100,000 to 300,000 people. It was the ambivalent response of West Pakistan to this appalling natural disaster (plus the ethnic, cultural and language differences between Pakistanis and Bengalis plus an unequal sharing of resources) that contributed to the success of the Awami League in the Pakistan national elections of 1970. A Bengali majority in the National Assembly insisting on greater autonomy for the East was not acceptable to West Pakistan and a nine-month civil war followed. After victory on 16 December 1971, a national government of Bangladesh was formed. The first general elections were held in 1973 and were won by the founding father of Bangladesh and Awami League leader, Sheikh Mujibur Rahman. However, following a widespread famine in 1974 (characterised by massive flooding as well as high mortality) plus violent insurgencies in January 1975, the Sheikh declared a state of emergency coupled with a switch from a parliamentary to a presidential form of government. This secularisation of government caused widespread dissatisfaction within the military and Sheikh Mujib along with most of his family were assassinated in a military coup (15 August 1975).

compromised (or so it seemed). As a young couple whose personal goals until then were measured by exam success, making a sporting team, achieving a career choice or coping with a failed relationship, being confronted with the rawness of a daily struggle to survive was something never experienced, let alone imagined.[5]

As I saw many times, thereafter, living in a gender divided society can sometimes be a leap too far, especially for women. Add to this their classification by the UN as "accompanying spouses", and you have a challenge. Local regulations often do not help. They can prevent a spouse from obtaining a working visa. The common accoutrements of expat life[6]—family, a social and sporting life focused on embassy clubs, volunteer work, cultural immersion and travel can prove insufficient substitutes for a person wanting proximity to the known, to family, to the pursuit of their own professional career. Alone, they are often left to manage as best they can. Add the traumas of transition and, as we discovered, many a UN couple live separately, punctuating absences by regular visits and, at that time, a weekly aerogramme. Not surprisingly, divorce rates are high among expatriate couples as each, in turn, navigates their way through the rigours of an international life.

In retrospect, my assignment to Bangladesh shows just how much emotional toughness is required when you move to a new house and country. Ask any service personnel or army "brat". When it is a developing country, one so unlike what you have known and well outside your comfort zone, a successful transition takes self-assurance, plus an outward focus that typically comes with work. But who am I to talk about successful transitions when, given my peripatetic life, I have never been very good at relocations? From my first boyhood camp through to changes of schooling, I have struggled with moves. Now, here I was in Bangladesh, charged by the ILO with piloting a project in a rural location. I may have been new, naïve, and emotionally challenged but I was committed and idealistic. I had to get on with it. But where to start? The local ILO office seemed to be the place to go.[7]

The country representative of the ILO was an English woman who had served most of her career in Geneva. She was steeped in the traditions of the agency, namely, its conventions and resolutions.[8] It never occurred to me

---

[5]Letter to parents, 6th August 1977.

[6]"Expat", short for expatriate, a term widely used in foreign communities the world over.

[7]Letters to parents, July 12, 1979.

[8]International labour standards, which are made up of Conventions, Protocols to Conventions and Recommendations are legal instruments drawn up and adopted by the international community. They reflect common values and set out basic principles and rights at work seen as critical to the ILO's constituents (governments, employers, and workers). Conventions are legally binding international treaties that may be ratified by the member states. Recommendations serve as non-binding guidelines.

then why her last posting was Bangladesh and why she had accepted it. She complained a lot about being there. Later, I would see such an appointment as typifying some UN assignments whereby a staff member was given a fait accompli. Leave the headquarters and go to the field or take early retirement. I didn't know if she fell into this category or not, but she and her husband had opted for Dhaka. When she retired she was replaced by another long- serving ILO staff member, this time a national of Bulgaria. Like his predecessor, he knew the system well and basically saw his role in terms of maintaining good relations with the labour ministry, plus the peak union and employer organisations. Neither representative ever came to see what one of their "experts" was doing in his rural posting of Comilla nor showed any interest to do so. Being a junior, it never occurred to me that they would not want to travel to visit my project. Nor did I anticipate receiving any briefing documents from them, any literature placing what I was to do in a development context (reference the Brandt timeline etc.) or any current or colonial history which, given recent military coups, would have been relevant. Consequently, I was not disappointed when none was forthcoming.

Representing UNFPA was an American doctor who approached her assignment with missionary zeal. In fact, she and her late husband had been missionary doctors in China before the communist takeover and she now brought that commitment to the UN.[9] Unlike the ILO representative, she came on a field visit to our project and chose to attend a village meeting. Dressing for the occasion in a sari, she lost her balance in the boat when crossing the river and fell in. With her sari floating about her, others jumped in an attempt to rescue her. She was pulled out and then sat, drenched, in the bottom of the vessel more embarrassed at the fuss she had made than the scare she had given. Later, her UNFPA replacement was another American who was less keen to be in the country but had a level of technical competence that saw him so frustrated with the UN that he left.

Unlike today, the journey to Comilla in the late seventies required being ferried across three very substantial rivers (the Meghna, Gumti and Dakati).[10] The one I remember most was the Gumti because of its proximity to Comilla.

Ratifying countries commit themselves to applying the convention in national law and practice and reporting on its application at regular intervals. The ILO considers it important to keep track of developments in all countries, whether or not they have ratified a convention or not. In this capacity, the ILO provides technical assistance if necessary. See Chap. 1, p. xx.

[9]After her retirement, her love of Bangladesh saw her continue on in the country as a volunteer until she returned to her Quaker roots and family in Pennsylvania.

[10]Most of the landmass of Bangladesh lies fewer than 10 metres above sea level with considerable areas at sea level. This leads to frequent and prolonged flooding during the monsoon season. With 700 rivers coming from the Himalayas the country is said to have a love/hate relationship with water.

This river originated in the north eastern hill region of Tripura state of India from where it followed a meandering course entering Bangladesh near Comilla District. About 135 km long within Bangladesh it had a strong current and during the rainy months its breadth could reach 100 m bank to bank. Flash floods were a common phenomenon of this river, occurring at regular intervals. So much so that until substantial flood embankments were built, the river was known as the "sorrow of Comilla town". Not surprisingly, we were often warned to be careful as we waited in a long line of trucks, buses, and sedans before going down the bank and boarding the ferry. Stories were told of crowded buses missing the plank onto the ferry and plunging into the deep and swirling river with the loss of many lives.

On arrival in Comilla in late 1976, then a town of 100,000 and now a city of 588,772,[11] we were initially accommodated in "*Rani Kuthi*",[12] a large rambling guest house fronted by a colonnaded entrance. Then and now it is the guest house for visitors to BARD (Bangladesh Academy for Rural Development—the Academy). It was once the home of Dr. Akhtar Hameed Khan, a revered Pakistani, largely responsible for the establishment of the Academy in 1959, which was now to be my working destination.[13] Rani Kuthi was located near to the Nazrul Institute which was dedicated to the memory of the Bangladesh national poet, Kazi Nazrul Islam. Nearby and visible from the guesthouse was the "*Dharma Sagar*", a large lake or *dighi* dug during the years 1714–1732 by a former King of Tripura[14] named Maharaaj Dharmamanikya. When we arrived we were met at the entrance by the housekeeper but apart from him there was no official welcome or any set of written

---

[11] "*World Urbanization Prospects*" UN Department of Economic and Social Affairs: Population Prospects, 2018.

[12] *Rani* meaning queen and *Kuthi*, house.

[13] BARD was formerly known as the Academy for Rural Development when it was established in 1959 prior to the independence of Bangladesh. What became known as the "Comilla Approach to Rural Development" was a unique approach to rural development conceived by Dr. Khan. In the Comilla Kotwali Thana, small farmers were organised into village-based cooperatives for the diffusion of modern agriculture technology with the aim of increasing productivity from the limited agricultural land. By the 1960s, these cooperatives had evolved into a federation known as the "Thana Central Cooperative Association". To those familiar with the agricultural development literature of the time, this 'Comilla Approach" was an important innovation and one that held great promise for the raising of millions out of poverty. So much so that through the support of Michigan State University, a substantial campus had been built to provide training for both official and non-official members of the public and private institutions working on rural development. The training was provided in the form of courses consisting of workshops, seminars, and excursions. Since its inception BARD has conducted a number of large and small scales development programmes.

[14] Tripura is a state in Northeast India bordered by Bangladesh (East Bengal) to the north, south, and west, and the Indian states of Assam and Mizoram to the east. The Bengali people form the ethno-linguistic majority.

instructions on how we were to proceed.[15] Again, I never saw this as a problem as, being inexperienced, I had no expectations. Later, I came to see it as the norm. Any briefing that you might receive was the exception. You were just expected to get on with it.

It was winter when we arrived. The nights were crisp, humidity was down, and the countryside was a mass of yellow mustard seed (*sarisa bija phula*). Mornings at Rani Kuthi consisted of drinking tea and an early lunch time *tiffin*[16] brought to us by the *baburchi* (Bengali for cook). We sat on wicker chairs in the winter sun watching the movement of people amidst the chaotic sounds of birds, roosters, fruit bats, barking dogs and the ringing of rickshaw bells. Voices rang out all speaking in a strange but increasingly familiar babble.[17] We saw the poor of the town come to complete their ablutions by standing on the steps leading down into the lake and bucketing the water over their heads while modestly keeping their *lungis*[18] wrapped around them. It was all very routine, rather sleepy in fact. No one seemed to mind anything— the dust, the noise and the perils of chaotic traffic. Even the teams of beggars, *fokirer dol*,[19] were given clearance as they dragged themselves through the town displaying their awful handicaps. Palms upraised, they recited verses from the Quran in the hope of receiving a sympathetic *taka*.[20] No one seemed to notice let alone protest that they gurgled, spat or urinated onto whatever wall they passed. Later, the number of beggars would escalate at the annual town exhibition where they lay in a clump, deposited there at the entrance or propelled themselves around on boards by using their cloth-bound hands to push their way along. At day's end you would still find them there calling out in the half light as the power dipped owing to the extra demands made by the ferris wheels and other entertainments.

At the guesthouse, we met another ILO couple, housed there while engaged on a separate project, one to do with public works. They were English. Having spent many years on the development circuit, far from home,

---

[15]Twenty-two years later when reassigned to Headquarters in New York, nothing had changed. There was no welcome then nor any briefing documents or guidelines for living in New York. I set out to change this.

[16]Tiffin is an Indian English word for a type of meal. It can refer to lunch or a light breakfast. It is derived from English colloquial or slang *tiffing* meaning to take a little drink. For us it often consisted of rice, lentils, curry, vegetables, chapatis or "spicy meats".

[17]Letter to parents, June 13, 1979.

[18]The *lungi* also known as a sarong is a traditional garment worn around the waist in India, Indonesia, Bangladesh, Pakistan, and Cambodia.

[19]A group of four or five beggars.

[20]*Taka* is the currency of the People's Republic of Bangladesh. The most commonly used symbol for the taka on receipts while purchasing goods and services is "৳" and "Tk". ৳1 is subdivided into 100 *poisha*.

they had adopted practices that brought order and familiarity in their often remote and isolated existence. These included sitting together for a shared drink in the evening, dressing for dinner, being waited upon by their *baburchi* and playing canasta afterwards, a rummy card game which they taught us to play and which we came to love. As for other foreigners in Comilla, there were very few. Closest to us was an American Catholic priest from the midwest who had been there for the last twenty years during which time he had ministered to a small community. Another was an evangelical Christian family from America of whom I only ever heard and never met. There were also some volunteers from the American Mennonite Christian community and a Japanese aid agency, JICA.[21] These were dedicated people focused on small-scale agricultural projects and the introduction of "appropriate technology" into traditional farming. After I had met them all, I did not quite know what to do next. I sensed I had to do something. I decided to leave the comfort of the guesthouse and its established routine, move to the Academy, and get started.

The drive from Comilla town to the BARD campus located at Kotbari, 10 km away, was along a narrow dusty road through open rice paddy. It wound past the remnants of an airstrip which the Japanese had bombed during the Second World War. Visible nearby was a Commonwealth War Cemetery where some 400 soldiers of British, Indian, Japanese, and Burmese origin were buried, having lost their lives on the Burma front during the war. Despite its remote setting, tourists came every year to visit this cemetery. Further along that dusty road, which I came to know so well, was the rather rundown Mainamati Museum. Located adjacent to excavations, it displayed historical artefacts from the seventh and eighth centuries. When we finally reached the Academy, we drove through a rather imposing arch marking the entrance and once inside entered a substantial campus of low storied buildings and long corridors. The campus was cordoned off. In a sense, it was a closed economy.

The BARD campus consisted of classrooms, conference rooms, a mosque, library, a health clinic, sports complex, and other amenities. They were all reached by external corridors. The staff housing was located off a semicircular road which followed the perimeter of the complex and along which staff would walk with their families in the cool of a late afternoon. Shady tropical trees protected them with a large part of the campus devoted to orchards, experimental vegetable trials, nurseries and park land. It was a secluded world unto itself. Outside the walls was another world of peasant farmers, verdant

---

[21]JICA stands for the Japan International Cooperation Agency.

fields and villages marked by thatch huts, their locations tagged by palm and coconut trees. The colour changed with the seasons: rice paddy in the humid monsoon, cloud build-up most days, and then sunflowers in the clear crisp winter days. Produce sellers lined the sides of the road at the entrance to the campus hawking their wares: fruits, vegetables, live chickens, a butcher chopping away a freshly killed goat on a rickety table (there was no refrigeration). Directly across the road from the BARD gate was the entrance to a guarded military camp: a *cantonment* where later I would be granted access to pass through on my way to Dhaka thereby avoiding the trip into Comilla town and out again.

The house allocated to us was one of four along a row. It was solid but modest and furnished with the basic necessities. In 1976 I felt it important that I live with my local colleagues (as distinct from a secluded compound), a conviction I carried throughout my UN career. To furnish the cottage, we bought cane chairs, jute carpets, a fridge, kerosene cooker and a small black and white television, the first I had ever owned.[22] There was no hot water. In the cold months we washed by standing in an iron bucket and ladling heated water over ourselves. What was critical were the ceiling fans and we quickly realised we needed to sleep directly under them, as they roared overhead, if we were to be free of the mosquitoes. If there was a blackout (a frequent occurrence), we joined others sitting outside on the street, no matter what the hour. In the absence of the rapidly circulating air it was simply too hot indoors as well as too infuriating having to fight off the mosquitoes. Through contacts we were able to appoint a cook and what a wonderful man he was. Abdul lived in Comilla town and commuted daily by bicycle. Each morning, on his way to us, he would stop outside the entrance to the Academy to purchase the day's meal from that row of rickety stalls. Often, he would buy a live chicken which he strung over the handlebars and later slaughtered on our back step. One of his specialities was chicken curry as was vanilla custard and a local breakfast variant of muesli which he mixed together daily—*kismis* (raisins) added to *chatu* (cereal mix). We also employed a *mali* (gardener) who came on weekdays and transformed a barren patch into a magical coloured delight. Initially, we thought to clear and tend to the garden ourselves but whenever we ventured outside neighbours would come to watch us. Such foreign behaviour was a source of pointing and comment, especially when it came to our clearing the open drains which ran down both sides of the house. This was simply not something householders did let alone academic staff. You employed a *jharudar* (sweeper). We quickly adopted the local practice and

---

[22]Watching the 8:00 pm English news was a must.

engaged a man specialising in this practice. Normality was restored and the source of curiosity subsided.[23] Later, both our cook and gardener moved with us when I was transferred to Dhaka, and when we left Bangladesh I was able to arrange employment for Abdul in Saudi Arabia.[24]

Soon after we moved to live at BARD, we were given a rude shock. On a cold night during our first winter, *miscreants*[25] (robbers) attacked the house of my counterpart. They were armed with submachine guns. They quickly dispersed but there was a panicked and noisy reaction from those of us who lived on the lane. Once it was confirmed that all were safe and that nothing substantial had been stolen (apart from gold jewellery and saris there was little else of value in most staff houses), people began asking who these people were and why the last house? Some said they were rebels attacking a government installation; others that they were members of a notorious gang known to be hiding out in the Chittagong Hill Tracts. Rumours hinted that the occupant of the last house was engaged in some nefarious affairs. Finally, when it settled down, the thought crossed our minds that perhaps they were simply robbers who had mistaken that house for ours. We nervously dwelt on how easily it could have been us. We were foreigners, recently arrived, accompanied by a household of possessions.[26] We never did find out who the *dacoits* were nor did we ever hear if they were apprehended. Until then, we had assumed we were safe living on a campus patrolled by *chowkidars* (security guards) armed with *lathis* (clubs).[27] After the attack, the Academy strengthened its security, and we were never invaded again.

When I arrived at BARD in 1976, the "Comilla Approach"[28] was still seen as one of South Asia's most promising rural development initiatives. However, it was generally acknowledged that with the departure of Dr. Khan,[29] the Academy and its accompanying experimentation had stalled. To me it was

---

[23]It was and is, a very Australian trait that you need to be self-reliant. If this entailed rolling up your sleeves at the end of a day's training and putting the chairs on the table, prior to sweeping the floor, you did it automatically. Similarly, if it came to be cleaning the drains at the side in a house, you found a shovel and got stuck into it. But this is not always a universal practice. There are those who are tasked with these specific undertakings.

[24]Our gardener went home to Comilla.

[25]A miscreant is an Indian English word for a criminal. In Comilla it was used along with the more common term '*dacoits*' which is a Bengali term for bandit the spelling of which is a colloquial anglicized version of a Hindustani word.

[26]Fourteen years later when we had just moved into our newly rented house in Accra, Ghana, we were again burgled. We had scarcely begun to unpack the multitude of boxes. Thieves are often well informed!

[27]Clubs, consisting of a heavy stick (often bamboo) bound with iron typically used by the police in the Indian subcontinent.

[28]See footnote #13.

[29]See page 5.

immediately recognisable that there was a languor to the ongoing work and that the staff were basically resting on an institutional reputation built during the sixties. BARD had become bureaucratised, lost its dynamic and was going through the motions. Still, an aging leadership, in some cases still yearning for the days of East Pakistan when opportunities were there for ambitious young researchers to explore broader horizons in West Pakistan, kept the Khan legacy alive and the institution ticking over. Outwardly there was research continuing whose aim was to collect socio-economic data for planning and project preparation. Not that I was ever briefed on this as I was never formally introduced to the faculty and welcomed by them. In fact, other than a meeting with the Director and his deputy (with whom I became close), I was left to my own devices to navigate my way around. Critical then was my relationship with my counterpart. "Counterparts"? What and who were they?

Under the ILO system of technical cooperation, project counterparts were typically employed by the host institution and took responsibility for the overall management and direction of a project, and for ensuring that all interested parties ("stakeholders" in today's development jargon) were involved. They were to take the lead in achieving project results by organising local support and inputs and, most importantly, ensuring long-term sustainability. Well, that was the theory. Did my BARD counterpart fulfil these responsibilities? No, not that he could not but it was simply not a priority for him. Bright, he had achieved academic prominence early via joint publications with an American colleague. After being awarded a scholarship to study at Michigan State University in the United States, he returned prematurely to BARD without completing his degree. An opportunity forgone such as this had stigmatised him. He was thin, stooped, a chain-smoker and, typically, would urge me to go on ahead without him. That became the pattern. I was basically on my own. When I arrived, I peppered him with questions. I was keen. The so-called "expert", needing to be tutored in the basics of agricultural cooperatives and local culture. He began by telling me about the cooperative association based at the *Thana Training and Development Centre* (TTDC) from 1962–63. It was to be the vehicle through which we were charged with introducing programmes of social change: the thinking being that if farmers could break with the perceived inevitability of fate through the introduction, and adoption, of irrigation, fertilisers, improved variety of seed, crop spacing, and basic mechanisation, all provided via the cooperative, they could also accelerate key social changes—literacy, nutrition, women's employment and, most importantly, birth spacing by family planning. Indeed, the three objectives of our collaborative project were population education, family planning motivation and delivery of birth-control services. While my counterpart and I always got on well that was about as far as any orientation went.

My actual education began on my very first visit to the TTDC Centre. I was asked to present certificates to the male trainees who had completed their training courses. I stood there as they came forward, right hand outstretched to shake theirs, certificate in my left ready to hand over. As I leaned forward to greet the oncoming graduate, my counterpart leaned in and whispered, "Don't use your left hand to present the certificate". I stopped in mid-action. He was right. Wise words indeed which I never forgot. In the absence of toilet paper, it being too expensive to buy, most people used their left hand to wipe themselves.

On my second day it was the women who were lining up to graduate. No shaking hands here, just the certificate to be handed over. As I stood there admiring the beautifully turned out graduates in their saris and best jewellery, I suddenly had a note thrust into my hand. It was a '*chit*'[30] from the general commanding the local military cantonment. He was urgently requesting my help with a cholera outbreak. I knew it was the end of the monsoon and that the rivers had swollen as they did every year from September through December. What I didn't know was that their muddy waters spilled into the sewers, drainage ditches and wells used for drinking water. There was now a crisis. It was the worst outbreak of cholera since records had been kept in the Comilla district. People were dying in large numbers. But what could I do? It was our project vehicle,[31] our driver and my presence as a UN official that was needed. In the absence of ambulances, we were asked if we could transport patients from village clinics to the hospital. Not for the first time it was assumed I was a medical doctor. I am not. But we carried the UN logo on our car which suggested we were official. Back and forth we went from the thatched huts which were the assembly points to which the mostly sick children and women had been carried, to the overcrowded hospital. When it came to decide who was to be moved, saved in fact, I watched the medical staff pinching the skin on a patient's stomach to see if there was any elasticity. If the skin bounced back, they had not entirely dehydrated and there was hope.[32] If the skin remained elevated, little could be done, and they were left. Once at the hospital, our patients joined hundreds of others lying on

---

[30] An Anglo-Indian term from the Hindi *citthi* or the Bengali *chirkut* meaning a short official note.

[31] Initially it was a canvas topped Jeep whose metal floor would become so hot, I would sit with my feet up on the dashboard. Later, we upgraded to a second-hand VW Kombi Van which seemed so luxurious and spacious.

[32] Victims can die of shock and organ failure, sometimes in as little as six hours.

rusted iron cots on a plastic sheet with a hole in the middle. Underneath was a bucket catching the diarrhoea. An IV pole balanced precariously between the patients dripped in the essential electrolytes. There the patients lay limp, ashen, dehydrated and barely conscious as their bodies poured out all its fluids to flush out the bacterium. Such were the numbers that they lay on the beds, between the beds, in the corridors and on the stairwells. Nothing had prepared me for this.

After the crisis had eased it was time for me to focus, really for the first time, on why I was there. I began by reading the history of Bangladesh, especially focusing on its recent development and demographic challenges. I read again of the struggle in 1971 for the newly formed state of Bangladesh to emerge from East Pakistan only to be faced, soon after, with unprecedented development and demographic challenges. I was struck by how the newly independent entity had a population of approximately 80 million and a total fertility rate of 6.5–7 births per woman. Given one of the highest child marriage rates in the world,[33] this meant the country would have more than 160 million inhabitants within a quarter of a century, thereby further straining its economic development and its political stability. I also saw in the literature how 90% of the population was rural with the majority of the population (80%) involved in the agricultural industry. Traditional methods of farming were said to be commonly utilized with human labour involved at every stage of the agricultural process.

When it came to family planning, the First Five Year Plan for West and East Pakistan (1973–1977) included a goal of reducing the total fertility rate by 20% through the distribution of contraceptives and family planning education for eligible coupes.[34] This was soon changed, however, by the 'founding father' of Bangladesh, Sheikh Mujibur Rahman (1971–1975), when he dismissed family planning programmes as irrelevant and needing to be de-prioritised. Following the military coup that led to the death of Mujibur and the months of political turmoil that ensued, Major General Ziaur Rahman became the 7th President of Bangladesh on 21 April 1977. It was because of Ziaur's concern about the overall size of population, the rapidity of its growth and how best to constrain it that his government, through its ministry of population control with financial backing from foreign donors, was now encouraging innovative approaches.[35]

---

[33]52% of girls are married before the age of 18 and 18% are married before the age of 15. http://progress.familyplanning2020.org/content/partnership#anchor-sub_chapters-125.

[34]Warren C. Robinson, Family Planning Programs and Policies in Bangladesh and Pakistan.

[35]None captured more the spirit of the times than the pioneering efforts of the Bangladesh Rural Advancement Committee (BRAC). I first encountered BRAC in Comilla town when I witnessed a semi-literate woman with six months intensive training, perform a tubectomy. The patient came

I then turned to the project document to learn more about the innovation sought. Unfortunately, it added little to the general narrative. It was generic and essentially a repeat of comparable documents used elsewhere although tailored to the general Bangladesh situation. I never knew who wrote it, but it lacked data, measurable outcomes and any sense of the rural environment in which I was to operate. But it was, after all, a pilot project and it was now up to me to figure out the innovation needed. I had to consider: where to start? From my attendance at the Thana Training Centre I observed that it was the same participants who kept presenting for training at the Centre, time and time again. Whatever the course content, they would be there dressed in their finery. Were these the elected leaders of the cooperatives? Were they paid to attend? Perhaps they were staff sent by the village committee? I began to question the validity of all this training.[36] What were the results? Importantly, what changed as a result of the training or was the training simply an end in itself, not giving rise to any action? I resolved to go to the village and find out. But first I needed some local staff to travel there with me and once arrived, to interpret, and by talking with people and not at them help me understand the cultural context. It was time to recruit.

The first appointment made was the project driver. Soon after my initial meeting at the ILO office in Dhaka, a tall distinguished man approached me. He explained in slow English that his ILO contract had expired following the completion of a project and that he was now looking for a new appointment. Hiring staff was something new to me but I was taken with his quiet dignity, the absence of obsequiousness and when I heard he was from Comilla, I immediately appointed him. It was the best decision I made. Over the next three years I spent hours with him—back and forth trips to Dhaka; village meetings day after day, night after night; in and out of the town. He was a wonderful man, the first of many project drivers I employed and came

---

from a nearby village and when she arrived was given a new sari which she was to wear on leaving the clinic. The room for the procedure contained only the basic necessities—an operating table, boiling water for sterilisation and a very limited number of instruments. The paramedic explained to me that the procedure was easy because rural women had no fatty tissue so that after the initial incision, finding and looping the tubes was relatively straightforward. I watched her carry out the procedure from beginning to end and when it was over, I watched the client recuperate and then climb into a rickshaw dressed in her new sari. Later evaluation of the scheme found that there were fewer postoperative complications with these practitioners than with doctors performing the same procedure. Perhaps it was that the more complicated cases were attended to by doctors, but the lesson was clear. Innovation, intensive training, support and reward, evaluation and scaling-up were the way to go.

[36] As did others. "We begin with a focus on the...undertakings of the Bangladesh (formerly Pakistan) Academy for Rural Development at Comilla, which has been in progress for more than 15 years. It will be shown that though there has indeed been a marked and sustained increase in production, not small farmers but large farmers have been the beneficiaries" Harry W. Blair "Rural Development, Class Structure and Bureaucracy in Bangladesh" World Development 1978. Vol. 6. 1, p. 65.

to know. He became my friend as did his wife and children. When I left Bangladesh, I saw to it that he had another UN contract by which he could continue to support his family as well as maintain his dignity.

Other appointments soon followed. First, came a male secretary, his gender being the norm for clerical appointments at that time—a religious man complete with beard and *tupi* (prayer cap) who used his shorthand/manual typing skills to copy Koranic texts as skilfully as he took my dictation. He was a user of *pan* and would sit there cheerfully chewing away his lips red with betel nut. Then there was our female field worker—a local widow of a school teacher who had a natural ability to communicate with village women as well as an extraordinary memory to recall what happened to the very day a year ago or five years ago.[37] She was a tiny woman who when I first met her astonished me by chewing on raw chillies as distinct from *pan*. Later, I learned that this was a local remedy to ameliorate the pangs of hunger.

Our final team member was a male field worker whose origins I never quite knew other than it was somewhere in local government. He volunteered to join us. What a gift he was. He had a natural way with illiterate people. He respected their position and could sit, talk and debate with the village men, including citing the Koran and the relevant hadiths[38] when necessary. Where appropriate, he could also refer to common agricultural practices to illustrate his argument. Typically, a meeting would end with heads nodding in agreement to the points he made.

My first excursion to a village was not exceptional as regards the location. It was randomly picked from a large list. But it was revelatory in terms of the lesson learnt. It was winter, that time every year when the rice from last year's harvest had run low but the new crop hadn't come in. For two to three months food had become scarce, incomes had dropped, and families began to skip meals.[39] We had driven out of Comilla town, along a series of dirt

---

[37]A characteristic not uncommon to illiterate or semi-literate people.

[38]A hadith is one of various reports describing the words, actions, or habits of the Islamic prophet Muhammad. Of particular significance to our village work were the insights of Al-Ghazali, a Persian Sunni theologian, jurist, philosopher, and mystic who was born in 1058, Tous, Iran and died on the 19 December 1111. He wrote a famous ethics textbook *Kimyaye Saadat* or Alchemy of Happiness. "According to Al-Ghazali, *azl* or withdrawal is not wrong or against the basic tenets of Islam as long as it is practised for a proper reason. He mentions three important reasons for the practice of family planning. 1. Financial loss due to the automatic liberation of a female slave in case she is impregnated by her owner. 2. Health and beauty of the wife and husband. 3. Emotional strain and fatigue which might be caused by having a large number of children and numerous pregnancies." Gavin W. Jones and Mehtab S. Karim, editors ISLAM, THE STATE AND POPULATION C. Hurst & Co., London 2005 p. 128.

[39]Not surprisingly, known locally as the 'lean season'. Robinson, Family Planning Programs and Policies in Bangladesh and Pakistan.

roads, then parked the car before being poled across the river to the rick-shaws that awaited us on the other side. The village was pointed out to us, a clump of palm trees and thatched huts, one of many that dotted the land-scape. The rickshaw-puller had mounted his bicycle and we had glided off through the carpets of yellow mustard seed so evocative of the Bangladesh national flag. When we arrived and alighted, we looked around expecting to be met. It was mid-afternoon, there was a weak sun, insects droned. It was very still. Apart from barking mangy dogs whom we had disturbed, there was nothing, no-one. Where was everybody? Had we made a mistake? When the dogs had settled to scratch and lick, much to our relief,[40] we went looking for our contacts. An old lady emerged. She explained that the men were out working in the fields and that the women had either travelled into town or taken the opportunity to nap with their children before preparing the evening meal. Better to come back at another time, she said, probably best at night because everyone is home in the evening. How right she was. Lesson learnt. You needed to go at night, after the men had come in from the paddy, had their "bath" (a wash by bucket in a nearby pond), been to the mosque, taken their dinner and then repaired to sit at rickety tables drinking tea and chewing *paan*. By this time, the women would have washed the dishes, settled the chil-dren, and gathered in the narrow alleyways abutting the village centre to chat and observe their men. And, so it began. Night after night we made that journey. Hundreds of them. With experience and following experimentation, we developed a pattern. Pick up the team at dusk in Comilla, take a road out of town, turn off onto an unpaved side track, be ferried across the river if that was required and then climb aboard a rickshaw to glide through the night towards some distant village. Once there, speak to gatherings however big or small. Later that night, home through the dark after dropping off our team. Throughout we were learning, finding out what mattered to rural people, their struggles, hopes and ambitions. Importantly, we were becoming familiar with the traditional culture—the humour, the analogies, the religious underpinnings, people's fears, and taboos. Patterns were emerging which we needed to understand, respect, and address. The villagers may have been illit-erate, but they were challenging us with their ingrained wisdom and canny insights. Rapport was building but if we were not to repeat mistakes from the past—provided we could find out what these were[41]—we had to find some

---

[40]Rabies was common in Bangladesh and the sight of any dog behaving erratically was bound to set the heart racing.

[41]A common failing in the development field is not knowing what happened earlier, what worked and didn't work or not finding out what was going on in a neighbouring district, elsewhere in the same country or internationally. Not surprisingly, mistakes are repeated, successes not built upon and approaches announced as innovatory when they may have experimented with years earlier. An

answers to the questions being posed and the logistics of night meetings. One was immediately obvious. We needed to train some other teams, important also if we were to localise.[42] We also needed to reinforce our messages in a way that was not dependent on our teams but was an established part of traditional village life. Something that was already there; a cultural reality that people had grown up with, that was both entertaining and informative. We decided to use *Jari Gaan*[43] to get our message across—a technique that had proved effective when BARD used it in the late sixties.

Jari Gaan is a two-way dialogue with musical and choral accompaniment. Indigenous to Bangladesh, it appeals to men and women alike. Because of its tradition, we were told that women were particularly keen and willing to get involved. Perfect, we thought, and a possible key to the programme's sustainability. Project funds were accessed, and I hired a group of travelling musicians, along with their folk instruments.[44] More funds were then found for transport, a vehicle was rented and they were underway. Night after night they travelled from village to village, arriving at sunset and instantly drawing a crowd. Like seasoned performers they used humour and pathos to entertain. It was the sound of the *dhol* that typically greeted us as we arrived in the village. Later, we wrote scripts for our *jari gaan* teams based on the exchanges we were having with the villagers and the questions they asked. Because language was always a challenge, we collected local colloquiums for inclusion, using everyday examples that people could identify with. Reinforced was the development mantra to "start with what you know and build on what you have".

Over time and largely through trial and error, we came to see that FP was not an alien topic to the villagers. After all, their own farming practices were predicated on spacing and the management of fertiliser and nutrition. They also knew about the practice of *azl*, a traditional form of contraception commonly known today as withdrawal.[45] But, not surprisingly, it soon became apparent that it was virtually impossible to expect that a conversation about contraception could be started between husbands and wives let alone

---

illustration of this was graphically displayed at a regional meeting of UNFPA representatives held some thirty years after I had left Bangladesh. Announced as a keynote speaker was a contracted 'expert' on the use of the media. Her ground-breaking innovation, she told us, was her use of traditional folk music as a means to promote behavioural changes. She clearly had never heard of our *jari gaan*. See next page.

[42] Now part of what is euphemistically known as 'building capacity.'

[43] Persian *Jari/zari* for lamentation and Bengali *gan* for song or song of sorrow. Most are based on legends relating to the grandsons of Muhammad and other members of his family at Karbala. The performers, who are male Sunni Muslims, work chiefly as farmers and go from village to village.

[44] Folk instruments like a *sarinda* (a stringed instrument played with a bow), the *khamak* (a one-headed drum with a string attached) and a *dhol* (a double-headed drum).

[45] Coitus Interruptus.

the most appropriate method negotiated. Family planning was viewed as a women's issue with the responsibility lying squarely on her shoulders (ironically without any autonomy to make decisions). Husbands were not only not involved, but also were not allying with their wives in accessing FP and health services. This gender demarcation, common to many societies, was a challenge we needed to face. What to do? Given the sensitivity of the topic, we knew that joint sessions of men and women was a near impossibility. But suppose it was clothed in a different format, kept within village tradition, and was not embarrassing. Could we explain the advantages of 'birth spacing' in terms of rotating crops, spacing seed, and nurturing growth? Could we address long-held superstitions by explaining how the reproductive system actually worked? We needed to find a way to broach controversial subjects that did not breach cultural taboos. But what were these taboos and superstitions? We went to see the local Islamic 'mullah' to find out where he stood on the issues. After listening to him we sought verification in the Koran and the Hadiths. When we were satisfied with our religious authentication, the next challenge was how best to communicate our findings. Our search led us to another traditional means of spreading news in rural areas that were both entertaining and widespread. It was puppetry accompanied by a form of musical interaction. With the support of an audio-visual adviser from the British Council we began moulding puppets. Regrettably, our initial efforts did not go well. Rats ate our finished papier mâché figures made of newspaper with corn flour as a fastener. Alarmed, we sought to protect them. After allowing for a new set of puppets to dry, we put them inside a wire net only to later see weevils emerge having burrowed their way out of our miniature humans. Very disturbing! We started again using purer ingredients but then the humidity brought fungus. Finally, using special chemicals and ensuring the puppets were bone-dry before painting over with oil paint for extra protection, we had workable models.

Our first performance with our new team was called "Changing Times", a simple story about a village family which highlighted conflict between the generations. A daughter-in-law is constantly ill due to having too many children in quick succession. An enlightened neighbour finally convinces the mother-in-law that the solution is family planning. With its time-honoured joys and sorrow, the theme appealed to men and women alike. We then moved on to producing "Amina's Road to Happiness" another simple story which emphasized the importance of spacing between births by using contraception. These puppet performances were such a success that we decided to turn them into a slide show using real people. The slides could then be copied and shown multiple times. Our first challenge was to find a young married woman to play Amina. We enquired among our villages until we found the perfect candidate. She was agreeable and a date arranged for the first filming. That was when her husband intervened. He refused to allow her to act in a production about family planning and to be photographed, a not uncommon response given the widespread belief that both were anti-Islamic.[46] This was a crisis for us. Our efforts in support of family planning could now, potentially, be portrayed not only as foreign intervention but contrary to Islam. Urgently we sought clearance from a number of Imams to allow our production to continue. Once given, we searched for another "Amina". A young widow was identified and after we again questioned villagers regarding their sensitivity towards any religious implications in our script, and confirmed they understood and appreciated the themes, production began. When finished, we duplicated the slides, dubbed in the audio and using our battery-operated equipment made multiple presentations throughout the Thana.

'Understanding Contraception' was our third series of slides produced. This time, contrary to what we were told was culturally unacceptable, we explained how the reproductive system functioned, how the various methods of contraceptives worked, what issues could arise and how to cope with them. Traditional methods of birth control were also discussed along with superstitions. Whether it was the men watching in the village centre or the women away to the side, we found that people had a thirst for this knowledge. It was always our *jari gang* or our slideshows or our puppeteers that set the scene for the structured but interactive discussion about family life and family planning that followed. Most villagers may have been illiterate, but they understood the implications. After all, they had been farming for generations and knew what was required to bring healthy progeny into the world and sustain it through life.

The response to our nightly village rallies was overwhelming. A demand for contraceptive services was created to which we now needed to respond. But before we tackled this second phase of our pilot came a salutary lesson. After months of attending village rallies our efforts had become so well known that the Permanent Secretary (PS) of the Ministry of Population Control and Family Planning (MPCFP) in Dhaka decided to visit and attend one of our night-time meetings. All went according to plan—the musicians performed, a large crowd gathered, and a commitment was made by the village to support family planning. The PS was impressed. The next day at a meeting of the BARD faculty along with a large number of local dignities, he made special mention of my efforts. I was very pleased and acknowledged the crowd's

---

[46]Conservative Muslims believe that if God created man in his own image, any attempt to produce an image of a man is akin to creating an image of God, which is an act of blasphemy.

applause. Not so pleased was my counterpart. He may not have been going to our village meetings, but he felt he had been toiling away for years without any senior government official ever visiting him let alone publicly praising him for his efforts. Now, here was this newly arrived foreigner receiving all these accolades while he was consigned to the margins! A gulf grew between us. Later I received reports of his commenting adversely about me in the corridors of the government in Dhaka. With the project surging forward, I needed to learn a key lesson. As a UN technical advisor charged with working within a local institution, I had to be in a support role, not a leadership one. Whilst it was true that the impetus came from our small team to which my counterpart was basically a bystander, rather than a participant, any public prominence received must be accorded to him. If the project were to continue after I left, it had to be cemented within BARD, led locally and neither dependent on UNFPA funding (foreign aid) nor me as a technical adviser. Lesson learnt; it was time to consider what the next phase should be.

We knew we had to respond to the demand we had created. Not to do so would leave thousands of villagers disappointed that a promised response to their needs had not been delivered. We brainstormed until it was agreed. The villagers should elect two of their own to represent them, a man and a woman, and it couldn't be the same privileged persons who seemed to be present time and time again at the Thana Training and Development Centre, irrespective of the course. The nominations now became a routine part at the conclusion of our village rallies. We then trained the hundreds of elected villagers for six months at the Thana centre. They came in for half a day once a week. Travel for them was not easy. It took time. We had to allow for that. Costs were involved. We had to allow for that as well. Time away also carried a price and so compensation was paid. In the scheme of things these were small amounts, but people were poor, desperately so, and although I was opposed to incentives it was government practice to pay them and we were pleased to do so. Every topic was covered. Contrary to what was presumed, we never found the villagers to be shy when discussing reproduction and sex. Rural people the world over have an earthiness to them. While a Bangladeshi women might be completely covered by her *burqa* (an outer garment covering the body and the face) or have only her face concealed by her *hijab* (a veil separate from the sari), it didn't prevent them from talking.[47] At the closing ceremony to

---

[47] I should not have been surprised. Muslim women in the village may have been illiterate or at best semi-literate, they may have been answerable to their husbands, their mother-in-law's and to the prevailing codes of conduct but to assume they had no power, was to underrate them. They sought and gained strength by collective action and our team were of the belief that if we could embolden them to the stake out a position that was in the best interests of themselves, their children and their families then we were giving them choices in their lives, something that everyone was deserving of.

the training, the graduate received a framed certificate, a specially built blue wooden box in which to house lesson sheets, locally produced posters, record books and three months' contraceptive supplies (pills and condoms). It was quite a day, especially for the women graduates.

Once the training was complete, and the nominee had returned to their village, it was critical that we linked them up with a regular supply chain plus a referral source if they were unable to respond to their client's needs.[48] It was their project. They owned it. But now they would have to deliver. We knew that over time reliability and convenience **within** the village were key. We foresaw that storage of contraceptives and disposal in what was basically a mud and thatch hut was going to be a problem. Similarly, confidentiality when dealing with other villagers who in turn needed their own privacy was going to be critical. And, what of the innumerable other challenges we hadn't even thought of? We were confident our worker, even if illiterate, could explain a method and its correct use. We also agreed they could distribute for free or for a cost, whatever was viable for them in the long term. But how to avoid creating another dependency layer, one that relied on foreign aid? Institutionalise it was our answer. Embed it within the government machinery so that it did not depend on UN assistance. We went to see the local ministry officials armed with a letter from the MPCFC Secretary in Dhaka. We asked that our trained network be integrated into the existing government-run family planning programme. Of course, they agreed. We had the letter of instruction from the Secretary! But we soon discovered that institutionalisation was easier said than done. Government workers did not go to the village. At least not to any of our villages, although official government reports spoke of thousands being trained and posted. In hundreds of visits, we never saw one. So, we introduced the villager to their government counterpart before the training finished. We tried to cement the linkage between them by drawing up formal agreements. Where we could not create a secure contraceptive supply link we turned to social marketing and Population Services International (PSI), an American-based NGO.[49] Not perfect but we couldn't allow a pool of unmet demand to disappoint and fester. Had

---

[48]Rather like the recommendation of a British magistrate in the nineteenth century who was posted to Bengal. I remember reading how he argued for a trained primary health provider being located in every village—an early version of today's "one-stop-shop" as far as basic health needs are concerned (source unknown).

[49]PSI had come to our assistance following disruption to the government contraceptive supply chain. It was rumoured that thieves had boarded a freight train transporting USAID supplied condoms from the port in Chittagong to Dhaka. I presumed the aim of the theft was to ship the condoms across the border to India and sell them for a profit (the belief that the foreign product was better than the locally made). No, I was told. Thieves melted down the latex here in Bangladesh, poured it into moulds in the shape of children's toys and then transported the products across the border!

we done enough? We did not know. Monitoring and evaluation said we were on the right path. We were learning by doing.

Over time we did see our "champions' at the village become part of the wider government programme. Not all but most. Family planning in our thana became routine. Because of its advantages, Depo-Provera became the preferred method. No-one but the client needed to know, it didn't have a use-by date complication and there was no disposal problem. After training, our village workers became adept at inserting it.

During the fourth year of the project, the government found the pilot to be successful and recommended its expansion through the Integrated Rural Development Programme (IRDP). This was in keeping with the BARD approach where findings were to be used for training and information materials by respective public bodies, the aim being successful replication throughout the country. Research could then be used to evaluate national rural development programmes either independently or jointly. My days as a rural-based field worker piloting a pilot project were over. My days as a manager were about to begin: bureaucracy in the heart of the capital.[50] Before this leap, there was time to go on home leave to Australia. This was the first of many home leaves I was to experience but it had a pattern that was to repeat itself over and over again. The culture shock after years spent in another country, albeit a very poor one, the constant rushing about to see family and friends and the professional appointments needing to be made with doctors, dentists, chemists, bank managers and estate agents (to name a few). Then there was the inevitable departure. Saying goodbye to parents at the airport was always a challenge and as they aged you were never sure when next you would see them or in what health condition they would be.[51]

After rural Bangladesh, Dhaka was raucous and lively. It was also much hotter. May and September were the worst months. May because it is the month before the monsoon and September because it is the month after. But 1980 was especially bad, not so much because of the incessant rain but because it was the worst drought for 70 years. Day after day of 100° heat and 100° humidity. This meant power cuts as the hydro system dried up. No electricity meant no fans. Fortunately, at night fewer interruptions enabled a run of the air-conditioners.[52] The repercussions of the drought were hard on

---

[50]Letter to parents, February 1st, 1979.

[51]One of many challenges faced pursuing an international career. Another major one for any two-career couple was choosing whose appointment to be accepted while the other's career remained dormant. Always a very difficult decision especially in a country where the accompanying spouse is denied a work permit. Inevitably, one of the parties has to give way and it is, typically, the woman.

[52]Letters to parents, April 28th, 1979.

everyone, particularly on the poor who saw prices soar due to crop failures.[53] During the Muslim festival of Ramadan,[54] July in 1980, our "bearer", the *bawarchi*, after fasting during the daylight hours would collapse in a stupor before reviving with his evening meal. I would sit in my office with the sweat dripping off my forehead and down my arms, onto the desk. I was now on the sixth floor of a building in the Dilkusha Commercial Area of downtown Dhaka. There, my three project staff members and I shared a large room. Apart from the desks and chairs, it was virtually bare. The walls were distempered, marked, and chipped. On one there was a Bengali calendar and parallel to it, a large hole papered over by a piece of butcher's wrap. A fan whirred constantly overhead. Outside the door of my office sat some 20–30 clerks who seemed to us to be mostly idle spending their time happily talking and moving about. A lone typewriter occasionally chattered but could hardly be heard above the incessant hum of voices- all of men. There were no filing cabinets in sight. If one was fortunate to have one, they came without the necessary trays and petitions. Mostly, they lay empty, although if you were a senior officer you could put something personal in them and by so doing, demonstrate your status. But there were files. After all, this was a bureaucracy. So, where were they? They were tied together with red string and piled on top of each other where they gathered dust, went mouldy and were eventually eaten by a variety of insects. But they did mark out your space. In the absence of anything project wise, or interest shown, we decided to take leave and go to Darjeeling.[55] The other staff went home to Comilla.

---

[53]Letter to parents, June 13th, 1979.

[54]According to Islamic belief, Ramadan is the ninth month of the Islamic calendar. It is observed by Muslims worldwide as a month of fasting to commemorate the first revelation of the Quran to Muhammad.

[55]To travel to the hill station of Darjeeling in the 1970s you needed a special pass which could only be issued at the famous "Writers Building" in Calcutta (now called Kolkata). In this enormous building were housed the administrators of West Bengal which, for a long time, had been the centre of the colonial administration until the capital was moved to Delhi in 1911. In the seventies it was in the hands of a Marxist-Leninist State government. When we sought our permits, you had to navigate your way through this giant anthill to the appropriate floor. Once there, you were confronted by masses of files located just above head height in a type of artificial mezzanine floor. These files hung, suspended in dust and cobwebs, with birds nesting among the forgotten pages of some report that a clerk from Dundee wrote about the export of jute from Bengal to Melbourne in 1883. Below the files sat hundreds of clerks, carefully guarding their fountain pens, a prestigious possession, and the accompanying blotting paper. As observed in Dhaka, most of these clerks sat idle. But there was always one besieged with work and surrounded by people begging for his signature. The others were more productively engaged in talking, noisily clearing their throats, spitting into the spittoon, and generally doing all they could to avoid the risk of doing anything. No work meant no questions, a far safer alternative! Once you had your pass, you made your way to the Sealdah Railway Station, one of the major railway terminuses serving Calcutta. There, you caught the Darjeeling Mail to New Jalpaiguri, 564 km away in North Bengal where you then boarded the Darjeeling Himalayan Railway for the final leg up into the mountains. Because it was a night journey we walked to the station as evening fell. To this day, I can recall students running along the pavement to position themselves

On return from India the project team reassembled and waited for the government go-ahead to applying our model to more thanas throughout the country. We waited, and waited some more, until it was announced that the Planning Commission, following a request from the ILO, would conduct an evaluation of our pilot project. The team agreed this was a sensible decision knowing that our efforts had been of limited duration and confined to only one area of Bangladesh. We looked forward to explaining our approach back home in Comilla. We awaited the Terms of Reference. When the Commission lost the project file and asked to borrow our files, we realised a start had not been made and that precious time had been lost. There was no choice but to laboriously type out our documentation backed up by carbon paper and assemble a new file. Once handed over, we awaited the outcome. Nothing! What was going on? Nothing, in fact. We all wanted to go back to Comilla. I wanted to be back working at village level rather than seated here in this stifling government building twiddling my thumbs.

Delays and more delays. The evaluation had been concluded, the results extremely positive, and a new project document written based on expanding the model we had developed. But it was yet to be approved by the government. All that was required was for the Secretary, Ministry of Local Government, Rural Development and Cooperatives to instruct a subordinate to issue a two-line letter approving the scaling-up. The Minister had signed off, we were told, but the Secretary's signature was still awaited. Now, however, there was a personal element to this approval. My ILO contract was due to expire.

---

under the streetlight where they were to spend the night doing their homework and later sleeping on their rolled-out mats. Crowds at the Sealdah Station were of an intensity that I had never seen before even in Dhaka which in the nineteen seventies still had provincial overtones dating from colonial times when Calcutta was the capital of Bengal state. When we arrived in New Jalpaiguri on the following day and after alighting, stood on the station awaiting our connection, I learnt a lesson I never forgot. I had leaned forward to see if our train was approaching and as I turned to my wife to tell her it was not yet in sight, I saw that our suitcase was no longer behind us. Frantically, I looked up and down the station. In the distance, and about to exit the platform, I saw a man heading out through the turnstiles carrying our suitcase. I shouted, took off and gave chase. He turned, saw me, dropped the case, and dashed off into the crowd. Relieved, I grabbed our belonging and clutching it to me returned to where we were standing and awaited the arrival of the train. There we stood for another half hour or so with the suitcase now in front of me. As we were about to board, we were interrupted when a policeman approached us with the information that the offending thief had been apprehended and was being held in the station lock-up. "Would I mind coming to identify him?" I agreed. When I arrived at the relevant office I was greeted by a gathering of concerned policemen and there at the centre of them was the offending miscreant. He was a slightly built middle-aged man who prior to my arrival, had obviously been given a beating. He stood there, downcast, holding his tattered shirt (*shabdkosh*) in his hands. "Was this the man and did I want to press charges?" I was confused not knowing what to do. Should I condemn this frail, now crying man? "Please don't," he said in broken English as if reading my thoughts. "I have been a thief on this station for 30 years and without the little money I make from thieving, I am unable to provide a decent dowry for my four daughters. Please sahib!" I agreed and returned to board the train.

It was dependent on there being a project. Only when the Secretary signed would the funding flow. Recall that these UN projects were tripartite undertakings (i.e. government as local implementer, UNFPA as donor and ILO as technical executor). We were all frustrated. Indifference, bureaucratic inertia, and domestic politics seemed to be winning.[56] No, said the ILO office in Dhaka, relax. These delays were quite common, they told us, they could go on for some time. As a bridging arrangement, they extended my contract by three months. I had no choice but to just sit and wait. I turned to other matters, matters more personal and longer lasting.[57]

Before arriving in Bangladesh, my then wife and I had come to the view that whatever number of children we might have naturally, we would also adopt an equivalent number. This was an ethical position not taken for practical reasons but rather one based on our understanding of a world divided into have and have-nots and a conviction that as affluent Westerners we had a responsibility to do what we could in sharing the load of the world's abandoned children. It was a position that demanded our doing something as distinct from just having good intentions. As a newly married couple, we had not necessarily thought through how our commitment might manifest itself, but on arrival in Bangladesh we were receptive to the idea of adoption should the opportunity present itself.

It was just after our arrival in Comilla that we met Father Dan Kennerk, a priest from Fort Wayne, Indiana, USA.[58] Father Dan was a long-time resident of Comilla and one of the few foreigners living in the town. When we mentioned to him that we were thinking of visiting Chittagong,[59] he suggested we stay with the Marist Sisters who had a convent there. In March 1977 we clambered into our Jeep and headed south-east out of Comilla along the Dhaka-Chittagong Highway. In the 1970s it wasn't the easiest journey to travel 140 km to the second city of Bangladesh. There may have been fewer cars than now but without air conditioning it was a hot and dusty journey in our old American jeep—so hot in fact did the car become that you couldn't keep your feet on the floor. I would sit there bouncing along with my shoes on the dashboard, knees under my chin and elbow resting

---

[56]Letter to parents, 21 December 1979.

[57]Included here was teaching my daughter to swim. In the absence of those night-time village meetings I now had time. In the early evening we would go to a hotel swimming pool (the same one we stayed in on first arrival in Dhaka). First, she held on grimly to my back as we went up and down. Then it was the shoulders, later an arm and, finally, alongside, with me keeping a watchful eye.

[58]Father Dan Kennerk, 1914–2001, is buried in Dhaka.

[59]The port city of Bangladesh and garrison town in the Second World War (despite an uprising against the British in 1930s).

on the open canvas flap that served as a window. When we arrived in Chittagong we went straight to the convent, a large red brick building adjacent to which was a school with an attached orphanage. The sister-in-charge took us straight away to meet the children, nearly all girls. Indeed, there was only one boy, a teenager whose life had been spent at the orphanage. We were told that boys, given their perceived value to the family no matter how poor, were rarely given up for adoption whereas girls were seen as a cost that could not or would not be borne.[60] They were of all ages, from toddler to teenager. Unlike today in Bangladesh, where it is forbidden that Muslim babies be taken to Christian orphanages, the children represented all castes and all denominations. They clustered around us, with the younger ones holding onto our legs and the older ones wanting to practise their English. We later visited the classrooms where the girls sang for us with the sole boy proudly displaying his language skills by translating. The sisters beamed but for them it was momentary relief. Given the numbers they had to care for, they were overwhelmed. Now, among their newly arrived charges, were four baby girls none more than two weeks of age. All were in a perilous condition. As we bent to look at these tiny infants, the sister-in-charge asked anxiously "Would you like to take one home?" Saving a life was her priority. "You can bring her back in six months if it doesn't work out." We looked again. "Yes, we will take a child, but which one?" We were asked to choose, and we did. Forty three years later and contrary to the oft-expressed response when hearing the story of my daughter, I have always felt I was the lucky one.[61]

The first six months for our new daughter were tough. Demand feeding, expert attention from the United Nations clinic in Dhaka and basic tender loving care (TLC) saw the baby thrive. In no time she transformed from a malnourished premature infant with a blood infection to a curly-headed chubby toddler. With the crisis past, the challenge now was to complete the formal adoption procedures, a process that required navigation through the Bangladesh and Australian legal processes. The sisters had rightly judged that we would not be coming back in six months, but they had not prepared us for the adoption minefield that lay ahead. Under Australian law in the 1970s, inter-country adoption was the authority of respective state governments. When it came to the State of Victoria, a court decision was required

---

[60]Traditional thinking said that boys could work in the paddy, earn income, and bring in a wife who would care for the parents in old age. Girls were only ever to be confined to the home and when given in marriage, required a dowry to be paid before they left to their husband's home.

[61]In 2008 my daughter and I returned to Chittagong and the orphanage. Although the city's Christian population was much diminished the Marist sisters continued to care for orphaned children, still mostly girls. We spent an emotional day there searching old files some of which dated back to the 1940s. Late in the afternoon we found the original documentation admitting my daughter to the care of the sisters. She was two weeks of age.

that an Australian birth certificate could be issued in the name of the child proposed for adoption. This, in turn, was dependent on a positive decision given by the agency responsible for intercountry adoptions, that the parents wanting to adopt were found suitable to do so. Interviews, questionnaires, and home visits were required before such a finding could be declared and for this you needed to be resident in Victoria. Once the couple were found suitable, a matching process would follow whereby a child would be matched to the couple. In our case, the child was already in our care before we could be considered as 'suitable' or not. The standard process had been averted. We were now required to travel home in order to place ourselves before the relevant authority to be evaluated. For that to happen, we needed a Bangladeshi passport to be issued in the name of our daughter, so that an Australian entry visa could be issued, and travel undertaken. This would have meant taking the local birth certificate to the office in Dhaka where passports were processed, pay the fee, collect the document, and then go to the Australian High Commission and apply for a visa. Straightforward? Yes, but there was a hiccup. The Bangladesh government was under such pressure from Muslim hardliners over Muslim babies going to Christian countries, that it had placed a ban on all intercountry adoptions. No passports were permitted to be issued. No passport meant no visa, which meant she couldn't leave the country which meant we couldn't leave in order to meet with the Victorian adoption authorities unless we left our daughter in Dhaka, something we were not prepared to do. Was this a Catch 22 situation? I didn't know but I knew we had to somehow break the impasse. We explored multiple options including crossing the border into India and then making our way from there. Finally, it was suggested that I make my case directly to the concerned Minister. An appointment was made, and I set out to meet him in the government offices. The government offices in Dhaka were then housed in a large imposing but rather ugly grey concrete building. Long external corridors led you down to the minister. Once inside his very large office, you were met with a cacophony of sound as groups of supplicants tried to attract his attention while others conducted separate meetings. In one corner, water was being boiled for tea on an open flame. In another, constituents from the minister's home electorate were sitting and eating amidst their voluminous luggage. Being tall, I stood out and immediately caught the minister's attention. "Come forward," he requested, "How can I help you?" I leant over the crowd gathered around his desk and explained my situation. Could he intervene by issuing an order that an exemption be made for my daughter to be issued a passport. He paused and thoughtfully considered the situation. "Why are you in Bangladesh?" he asked. I explained that I was with the United Nations working on a village-based project in Comilla. He paused again. "The UN, you say. I would certainly like a project similar to yours based in my electorate. Why don't you arrange that and then I will consider your application?" I was dismissed. What to do? I had little idea how to consider his request. I knew what he proposed was corruption, but we were in an increasingly difficult situation. We had to leave the country, travel to Australia and be interviewed by the relevant adoption authorities. I also knew that UN/Government agreements took years to negotiate and that ours in Comilla was part of a five-year UNFPA programme of assistance. Any addendum to that involving a specific district would take months to haggle over and, even if agreed to, would require supplementary funding. It was never going to happen. I needed to go back and see the Minister, be candid about his request and call upon his mercy. When I did so it was the same crowded office, the same groups of men trying to attract the Minister's attention and the same minister doing deals and giving orders. As was the case earlier, he called over to me and greeted me amicably. "How did it go with my request?" I apologised and explained how it would not be possible to meet his requirement. He took it with great equanimity. He was unfazed. "Where did you say you were from?" "Comilla," I said. "No, no, what country?" "Oh, Australia." The minister paused, as he had done earlier, and considered this new piece of information. "I would certainly like to go there. See what you can do." This time I had the chance to speak. I tried to explain that I had no connection with the Australian government and was simply an Australian national employed by the United Nations. It was no use. He could already see himself watching the play at the Melbourne Cricket Ground. I made my way out escorted by his smiling office boys. We were again trapped. The only option now was to make an appointment and go and see the Australian High Commissioner.

The Australian High Commission was located on a floor in a hotel in the Motijheel Commercial District. This was in the heart of the city, the business and commercial hub as it still is today. The High Commissioner was a senior diplomat with many years of experience. He gave me a very sympathetic hearing. After listening to me, he genuinely felt for my dilemma, but he could not, nor ever would, countenance such a blatant piece of exploitation. The minister's request was completely unacceptable. The High Commissioner was right. From the Australian perspective, nothing could be done. We were stuck. I had no option but to return to Comilla.

Some months later, I discussed our situation with the Director of the Academy. Could he advise me? Was there some way out of this impasse? Not really knowing what to do, the Director suggested that I see a former

Director of BARD who was now the Minister for Agriculture. This was a technical appointment, the Director explained, not a political one. As such, he surmised, you may avoid all the wheeling and dealing. Moreover, this minister was senior in the cabinet hierarchy to the Minister for Social Welfare. That did it. I made the appointment and headed back to Dhaka. Unlike my earlier visits to the Secretariat, I found my meeting with the Minister for Agriculture surprisingly different from that with the Minister for Social Welfare. To begin with he sat alone at his desk.. No one else was present. He invited me to sit down. Secondly, he heard me out, silently reflecting on what he might do. I waited. Finally, he opened a drawer, pulled out a pad embossed with his name and ministerial portfolio, and hand wrote a message in Bengali. He then instructed me to, "Take this *chit* to the Minister and give it to him." With that, I thanked him and left not knowing what he had written but I thought it best to have it translated before I again visited the Secretariat. I took it to the officer in charge of intercountry adoptions. Over time I had come to know her well as I sought to navigate the bureaucracy. She, like many others, was deeply disturbed by what this embargo was having on the number of orphaned and abandoned children involved, and on their prospective parents around the world. She read the chit. As far as I could tell it was only a few words. "This is wonderful," she exclaimed, "He's requesting the minister to grant an exemption so your daughter can be issued a passport. On this basis we might be able to have all the children released!" All the children? What children were these? These were the 100 or so children who had been promised to parents in western countries but owing to the embargo were languishing in shelters around Bangladesh. They were all on a list now being held out to me. "You can take this to the minister and have him sign it." I recoiled. No way. I was not interested in any list. I was only interested in one case for which a handwritten *chit* might now break an impasse. I was not going to risk the future of my daughter on the basis of countless others with whom I had no connection. The pleading went back and forth. What if the minister saw through the ruse? What if I incurred his wrath? What if he wanted an even bigger deal? No, it's easy for you, came the retort, your child is with you. Think of all those anxious parents waiting for their child now deteriorating in substandard care. What a dilemma! Finally, it was agreed. I would take two lists. The first was a two-page list of names who had been cleared for adoption and included among them would be my daughter. The second was specific to my daughter's case and her case alone. Back I went to the minister.

It was the same scene as it had been on the previous two occasions only now it was winter, and the *peons* had changed into their heavy-duty cotton uniforms. There were the usual crowds making the usual noise over the usual deals being done. The kettle boiled in the corner and an overflowing cup of tea complete with powdered milk and sugar was thrust into my hand. I edged forward to catch the minister's eye. He saw me and after a cheerful welcome asked if I had managed to arrange his trip to Australia. I apologised, explaining that I had seen the ambassador and it was simply not possible. Hesitatingly, I then passed him the *chit* and the two pages of names pointing out where my daughter's name was. He read the brief note, instantly asked for a pen which I immediately handed to him, signed and stamped both pages. All 100 names were released. He had unwittingly signed away all of them. I thanked him and left hurriedly. Back at the office for intercountry adoption the signed document was a cause for celebration. Adopting parents could now make their travel arrangements. Transport could be organised to bring the children to a central location in Dhaka where they would meet their new parents before travel. For my wife and I our personal nightmare was over. We had the birth certificate and on the basis of the minister's signature, we now successfully applied for a Bangladeshi passport. Once given, the ambassador himself issued the visa. 40 years later, that passport is amongst my daughter's most valued possessions.

Meanwhile, back at the 'front line of development' or rather the backwater of bureaucratic inertia, we were learning how pilot success can be stifled by an insistence that it be replicated. We were caught between donor and recipient. Locally, there was little interest for what was, basically, an external requirement—expand the pilot project. In retrospect, I should not have been surprised. The need of agencies, such as the ILO, to chalk up funding, the push for donors, like UNFPA to spend and the welcoming hand of Bangladeshi bureaucrats, keen to take whatever was offered to them, often resulted in delays, underspending and only lip service being paid to meeting the needs of the most deprived. And, so, it would have continued until either I became fed-up or the funding was withdrawn. Unexpectedly, though, a 30% cutback in global funding to ILO from UNFPA decided the matter. The first of many oscillations in US funding to UNFPA resulted in reduced country allocations and the ILO team in Bangkok withdrew many of their in-country advisers. No contract meant either repatriation to Australia or reassignment elsewhere. As I contemplated my future, the long-standing links between the leadership of the Bangkok Team and Sri Lanka (the team leader was from Sri Lanka) provided an option. I was transferred to Colombo.[62]

---

[62]During the period of uncertainty when it was not clear what would happen, an old UN hand suggested I push for any one of the following three countries: Liberia, then a dictatorship but a settled one and economically said to be in the hands of the Firestone Tire and Rubber Company;

When I left Bangladesh, I never pushed to determine what would happen to "my/our" project in Comilla. I should have. I naïvely hoped our team was now sufficiently institutionalised in the rural government fabric that it would sustain itself. But the absence of any interest by IRDP to support the model let alone expand it, did not bode well. A report prepared by the Ministry of Health and Population Control containing a list of the UNFPA-funded projects, 1984–85, vindicated my pessimism.[63] There were only six. Our project in Comilla which was alive and active only four years earlier, was not one of them. Was the explanation the continuing financial cutbacks? Perhaps the project lacked priority, being rurally based and out of sight of the urban organised sector? Maybe I hadn't advocated strongly enough for it? Maybe my experience just typified short-term foreign aid projects whereby an initiative is proposed by an external donor, passively accepted by the government and ultimately dependent on an external driver, in this case, me? Good intentions coming to naught without government buy-in. It wasn't self-sustaining after all or so I thought (meaning, in a perverse sense, now that I had another posting, I was the ultimate beneficiary of my own efforts). But then in September 1985, five years after I had left, LAPTAP announced approval by UNFPA of a Family Welfare Education and Motivation for FP services through Rural Development Cooperatives. Implemented in 30 upazilas in the vicinity of three rural academies including BARD and other cooperative colleges and institutions, it aimed to work through cooperative office bearers, utilising an "approach tested and proven during the implementation of an earlier pilot project."[64] 100,000 members and their families in 2,250 cooperative societies were targeted via our programme model. Emphasised was the usage of existing institutions with national staff providing the day-to-day implementation. We were not forgotten after all. They were building on our efforts. It was a massive endorsement. Was the new project a success? Did the teams still go to the village or did they confine themselves to an office in the town? Were our varied entertainments still enthusing villagers? Was the training given a measure of an activity having taken place and money

Afghanistan, another dictatorship but with a mountain climate and a small middle-class capital; and, for something culturally different, Sanaa in Yemen, safe because it was in the grip of the authoritarian government.

[63] Ministry of Health & Population Control, Population Control wing, Government of the People's Republic of Bangladesh, "Population Control Programme in Bangladesh: Past, Present & Future" 1986, page 31.

[64] "UNFPA Approves Six New Projects" in LABOUR AND POPULATION ACTIVITIES IN ASIA AND THE PACIFIC, Published by the ILO Labour and Population Team for Asia and the Pacific, September 1985, No. 21.

spent or was it followed up to reinforce behavioural change? Had contraceptive supplies kept up with the demand? Regrettably, I do not know the answers to any of these questions.[65] The project was announced after I had left Bangladesh frustrated that our proposed expansion was stalled in the government bureaucracy. It was an example of how projects stop and start and of how external assistance even when as modest as ours, can be cut and then restored.[66] By 1985 I had lost touch, as the typical 'expert' often does, and moved on.[67] For me, Bangladesh was now not only my first UN assignment but the source of a life-changing relationship—one between a father and his daughter.

---

[65]Although, in retrospect, I like to think that Bangladesh's later success in reducing population growth owed something to our efforts; that the institutional links we established between the departments of health, population control and village cooperatives were sustained.

[66]Nearly 40 years later I read of a project being funded and executed by UNICEF. Based in Dhaka it sought to bring family planning to villages via traditional institutions like cooperatives. Did the international expert know of our experiences in Comilla? Did he/she know what other agencies were doing in the field of family planning or had done? I doubt it.

[67]Today, 2021, Bangladesh is booming. It has come a long way from the terrible poverty that I witnessed during the late seventies. Recent economic growth has averaged around 6% per annum and, with a population approaching 165 million, Bangladesh is one of Asia's major economies. Classified as a middle-income country, its life expectancy at birth (72 years) and low population growth rates (1.34% in 2017) place it ahead of India.

4

A Success?: Sri Lanka

They were very good years until it was all over

I would like to say I made a difference in Sri Lanka. I didn't. My counterparts did. Because of them I choose to write about a country I enjoyed immensely. My appointment there was a continuation of an earlier ILO proposal to UNFPA that a series of projects be initiated aimed at improving the population education of industrial workers via influential cadres such as trade union secretariats and labour leaders.[1] Accordingly, my portfolio of project responsibilities in 1981 covered workers in the plantation sector (coffee, tea, and copra), the rural employment sector, and the urban labour sector.

I was assigned to the Ministry of Labour where two ILO 'experts' had preceded me. Unlike Bangladesh, I was no longer piloting a project in the rural areas, alone and learning by doing. I was an advisor to a well-established programme.[2] During this time the ILO had trained three ministerial counterparts and when I arrived these three were not only fully operational but a pleasure to work with.[3] I was told one was a Tamil, another Sinhalese and third a Burger. Initially, this meant nothing to me, although later I came

---

[1] "Rafael M. Salas, op cit p. 45???).
[2] Letters to parents, 2 May 1980.
[3] Letters to parents, 21 December 1979.

to understand the language, religious and historical differences.[4] Together we travelled the country enjoying the hospitality of the provincial labour commissioners. In this way my two years' experience in Sri Lanka was not that dissimilar to multiple other international advisors before and since. Given the capacity of the Sri Lankans, they reflected the reality that I had little to add and more to gain.[5] Since 1974 the Ministry's efforts had reached 100,000 workers and provided family planning training to over 1,000 tea, rubber and coconut trade union representatives. Not surprisingly, with such a record, it all began uneventfully. After leave in Australia we were on our way. Orientation in the ILO regional office in Bangkok, and then the sub-regional office in New Delhi, followed.

Flying to Bangkok for briefing in the company of a three-year-old was now a question of navigating taxis, customs and passport control while carrying suitcases and those essentials needed to keep a toddler entertained. But people liked to help, especially, fathers with baby daughters. Would it be the same for mothers? Probably not. Such experience meant my respect for mothers bringing up children on their own went up a thousand-fold. Like them, I also took risks. I had to. I was back into the swing of being an ILO expert on the move. Briefing was set for Monday at the ESCAP building. But lest I became too smug, no one had advised me in response to my cables that Monday was an ILO holiday. Consequently, when I arrived at the ESCAP building, rested after the flight and spick and span in my office clothes, I was surprised to be greeted by a closed and unlit building. Puzzled, I enquired of the blue-helmeted UN security officer. He told me to come back tomorrow. Any briefing would be scheduled for Tuesday and Wednesday. I came back the next day, greeting the security officer like an old friend.

After the many so-called briefings I have attended over the years, this one followed the usual pattern. Colleagues mostly talked about themselves rather than focused on the specifics of the assignment, nor did they answer the questions put to them by the newly appointed staff member. Perhaps that is universally the case, public or private sector. I saw the same tendency on interview panels. No matter how many times you told the panel members to ask their question and then say no more as they awaited the answer most would continue elaborating on their question, providing options and then telling the candidate some anecdote from their own career. But I digress, it was on to Colombo.

The early eighties were a calm and peaceful time in Sri Lanka or so it appeared. Power seemed to have alternated between ruling families, the

---

[4]Just as I didn't know the ethnic differences some years later when I arrived in Kenya.
[5]As evidenced by the number of the international posts they went onto hold in the UN system.

Jayawardene's or the Bandaranaike's or the Senanayake's, and there was no talk of the Tamil Tigers.[6] In fact, when I was questioned by an Australian Tamil as to whether I had heard anything of the disgruntlement of his community, I was surprised and calmly told him I had not. When it came to politics, what I heard was the ongoing incredulity of the middle-class that their privileged youth had in 1971 sought to rebel against them. Although a distant memory, people were still baffled as to why their children had become so involved, they would take up arms. They had joined the Sinhalese Janatha Vimukthi Peramuna (People's Liberation Front), often abbreviated as JVP which was a Marxist–Leninist political movement that launched two armed uprisings against the ruling government.[7] The rebellion was bloodily suppressed with the loss of 30,000 youth lives.[8]

Those early days of mine in Colombo saw me fully occupied with settling into a new environment. Fortunately, my ILO predecessor had arranged a small flat for my daughter and I to occupy on arrival pending finding something more permanent. But being responsible for a small child meant I had to find suitable accommodation quickly along with day care. International consultants often talk about the challenges they face after office hours when confined to the loneliness of a hotel room. Now, I felt overwhelmed by the challenges of simply being new. I knew I had to avoid long hours on weekends sitting in a room with a toddler. I needed to find out about long term rental properties and figure out suitable locations (in the absence of any UN documentation on where you went or how you got there and whether there would be someone to go with you). Government colleagues were sympathetic but the divide between the foreigner, and their requirements, and local life styles, meant those colleagues didn't always know about rental opportunities in suburbs other than there own.[9] So, pending the signing of any rental contract, plus the arrival of my niece from boarding school in India

---

[6]From 1983 until 2009 a war was fought between the Liberation Tigers of Tamil Eelam (Tamil Tigers) and the Sri Lanka government. In its final weeks, around 40,000 mostly Tamil civilians were killed, bringing the war's total toll to more than 100,000 from a population of around 20 million. The Tamil Tigers were completely destroyed in 2009. The war was noted for its bitterness, with the Tamil Tigers using suicide bombing as a tactical weapon, as well as for targeted political assassinations. India intervened in the war in 1987. In retribution, a Tamil Tiger suicide bomber assassinated former Indian Prime Minister Rajiv Gandhi in 1991.

[7]The second was in 1987. Sri Lankan friends then wondered aloud if their country would ever achieve national unity, would ever rise above ethnic distinctions, and would ever move beyond a political system where the winner took all. Radicalisation of the marginalised seemed to have become the norm.

[8]Although the insurgents were mostly young, poorly armed, and inadequately trained, they succeeded in seizing and holding major areas in southern and central provinces of Sri Lanka before they were defeated by the security forces. Later they joined the government.

[9]Letters to parents, May 2, 1980.

at the end of her secondary schooling, and the shipment of our container from Bangladesh, I enrolled myself and my daughter into a hotel sports club, complete with pool, playground and expansive garden.[10] Not for the first time did I begin my background reading on population and development with one eye on a playful child, the other on the text.

The story of family planning in Sri Lanka is one of remarkable success, often cited as a voluntary alternative to that of the mandatory Chinese programme. In the debates over 'successful' programming, it is worth recording. It began with feminist pioneers before independence in 1948. Following their concern at the number of undernourished babies, the first clinic was opened in 1932. 1949 saw S. W. R. D. Bandaranaike, the inaugural health minister, call on the United Nations to address an 'increasingly urgent world problem' through birth control.[11] It was during his second term, 1956–1959, by the then Prime Minister, that an agreement was signed between the Swedish and the Ceylon governments to support pilot family planning projects. In history, this can be considered one of the first instances of bilateral assistance for family planning activities. Because the consensus among government officials was that population growth was detrimental to economic development, this consideration was incorporated into the 1959–1969 10-Year Plan.[12] To support a reduction in the growth rate, the government decided to experiment in areas consisting of predominantly Buddhist Sinhalese working in the rice, rubber and coconut industry, and to undertake similar experiments in those areas where, primarily, Indian Tamils, mostly Hindus, were employed in the tea industry.[13]

After the elections in 1965 that saw Dudley Senanayake elected as Prime Minister, the family planning pilot projects were extended nationwide. The goal was to reduce the birth rate from 33 live births per 1,000 population to 25 per 1,000 in 8–10 years. In support, the agreement with the Swedish was renewed in 1968. But it was a low-profile government effort because of fears that some among the Sinhalese saw the existence of family planning as

---

[10]As a result of this experience, joining a gym on arrival at a new posting became a regular practice of mine as I sought to adjust to a set of changed circumstances. Not only did it help with the mind/body conditioning but it also served to introduce me to a wide range of people outside the office context.

[11]Wright, N. H, 2007, 'Early Family Planning Efforts in Sri Lanka', in Robinson, W. C, & Ross, J. A, eds., THE GLOBAL FAMILY PLANNING REVOLUTION: THREE DECADES OF POPULATION POLICIES AND PROGRAMS, The World Bank: Washington D.C., p. 341 http://sitere sources.worldbank.org/INTPRH/Resources/GlobalFamilyPlanningRevolution.pdf [6 June 2015].

[12]Ibid. p. 343.

[13]The first experiment took place in Bandaragama, near Colombo, with a population of around 7,000 mostly Sinhalese Buddhists, and the second in Diyagama, with a similar population of predominantly Indian Tamils, with illiteracy rates of 20% and 75% respectively.

threatening their race, despite the existence of data that suggested no such thing. There was also some opposition among the Catholic community.[14]

In 1970, Sirimavo Bandaranaike came to power. The government reiterated its support and commitment to family planning. This time, no demographic targets were set. The existing Family Planning Bureau created in 1969 was integrated into the Maternal and Child Health Bureau, later named the Family Health Bureau. In came a new team of project leaders strongly committed to improving field performance, increasing field visits, inspections, and implementing a more rigorous system of fines and transfers as punishment for deficiencies. 1970 saw a United Nations mission visit Ceylon to plan further programmes with the World Health Organisation as the executing agency, and the UNFPA as the primary funder, specifically to a programme of strengthening medical services and their ability to provide clinical and contraceptive services, including the expanding use of sterilization.[15]

UNFPA sent in its first needs-assessment mission in 1973. As a result, a new Projects Implementation Committee was instituted with the Secretary of the Ministry of Health as the chairman; later, in 1974, this role was passed to the Secretary of the Ministry of Plan Implementation. This Committee was responsible for the coordination and evaluation of all population and planning activities, even those outside the UNFPA scope. UNFPA began funding in the following year with a $6 million programme. The nationwide effort to promote family planning led to an increase in the demand for sterilizations with the number of tubectomies doubling in 1974 and vasectomies increasing from 10 to 17%. Condom marketing increased using IPPF funds. The Population Services International (PSI) increased their use of mass media. By June, over 2.7 million condoms had been sold. For the first time in Sri Lankan history, condoms were marketed through non-clinical sources, such as boutique stores and grocery outlets. 1974 saw a new plan for contraceptive pill diffusion, with a cycle of pills costing only 75 cents.[16] In the same year, the rate of population increase dropped to 1.8%, marking the first time the natural rate of population increase dropped beneath 2% per annum.

---

[14]It became evident by the end of 1968 that the 1976 target would in fact not be reached. Instead a more realistic goal of 1 million family planning users by 1976 was pursued. Staffing issues had to be addressed and clinics, which had fallen behind in their services, needed to be improved.

[15]Yapa, L. & Siddhisena, P, 1998, 'Locational specifities of fertility transition in Sri Lanka', GeoJournal, Vol. 45, p. 179, Dordrecht: Kluwer Academic Publishers p. 253.

[16]Wright, N. H, & Fernando, A. J, & Herath, S. Y. S. B, 'Sri Lanka', Studies in Family Planning, Vol. 6, No. 8, Family Planning Programs: World Review 1974, August, p. 258, <JSTOR> [8 June 2015].

Of particular significance to the success of family planning programme in Sri Lanka has been the role of free healthcare. By the late 1960s free healthcare had been available for more than 15 years. Such care played a significant role in tackling malaria, infant and maternal mortality, and increasing child immunizations and feedings. Combined with free education, free to the tertiary level since the Second World War, Sri Lanka enjoyed some of the highest levels of human development in Asia.[17] By 2000, Sri Lanka had a total literacy rate of 90%, showing the huge role free education has played in Sri Lanka's development success. Access to education for women also played a key role in the success of family planning initiatives, largely attributable to those elements of Buddhist culture, which held women in high esteem.

Mass media also played an important role in the diffusion of family planning knowledge, through the extensive reporting of UNFPA activities notably the celebration of World Population Year,—special features and a number of editorials rolled out in 1974 regarding family planning and population issues. Other departments involved carried out extensive information campaigns, with content related to family planning included in bulletin posts, print articles, short films and even an essay competition.

In 1977, a new government headed by J. R. Jayewardene reiterated its commitment to family planning. He made a number of speeches, including one address to the 1979 Colombo International Conference on Parliamentarians on Population and Development. In his address Jayawardene stated,

> Our 'population explosion' is due mainly to something in which our people should rejoice. Our people are living longer than before.[18]

The President then went to say that he expected Sri Lanka's population to be 22 million by the end of the century. While acknowledging the contribution public education and health programmes had made to family planning

---

[17]The social philosophy of Buddhism has penetrated almost all aspects of Sri Lankan society, and the Buddhist enhancement of the female role on society can be dated as far back as 288BC, when a Buddhist order of nuns was established. Organised education also has a long history in Sri Lanka, dating back to the 3rd and 4th centuries BC, with the social value of education traditionally held above that of wealth in Sri Lankan society. Free and public schools began in their modern form under Dutch colonialists, but can be more closely tied to British legislation in 1830, which introduced legislation for compulsory education. Wright, N. H, 2007, 'Early Family Planning Efforts in Sri Lanka', in Robinson, W. C, & Ross, J. A, eds., op cit p. 341.

[18]J. R. Jayewardene, 1979, 'President Jayewardene on Sri Lanka's Population Policies and Programs', Population and Development Review, Vol. 5, No. 4, December, pp. 743 <JSTOR> [8 June 2015].

and population control methods,[19] his remarks highlighted the conundrum between the rapidly decreasing death rate, which occurred after independence, and the absence of a corresponding decrease in the birth rate. From 1948 to 1978, the population had doubled. It now stood at 14.5 million and was growing at 1.8% per year. One of the President's main concerns was the availability of land, and the potential consequences of serious shortages if population growth continued without further intervention. Following a second UNFPA needs assessment mission in 1980, the programme of sterilization[20] and contraception diffusion continued. Success came quickly. By 1987 a contraceptive prevalence survey showed that 62% of married women of reproductive age were practising a method of family planning, with 30% protected by sterilization, 39% of all women of reproductive age using a modern method of contraception and a further 23% practicing more traditional methods. When contraceptive prevalence was first estimated in Sri Lanka in 1969, it was estimated that only 5–6% of women were using contraception. When I arrived the programme was an unrivalled success.

By 1990, China and Sri Lanka had the lowest Total Fertility Rate(s) (TFR) in the World Bank's classified 'low-income countries'. They stood at 2.5 and 2.4 respectively, far below the average of 3.8 for comparable nations. In the same year, the TFR for sub-Saharan Africa was a staggering 6.5.[21] By 2006, Sri Lanka's population stood at 19.9 million, beneath the 22 million projected by Jayawardene. The TFR stood at 2.0, just under replacement rate. Life expectancy at birth in 2006 stood at 73 years, and infant mortality was 11.2 deaths per 1,000 live births. 70% of eligible married couples were practising some form of family planning, with 50% using modern contraceptive methods. In retrospect, while family planning programmes made much progress in achieving the demographic change in Sri Lanka, much credit now needs to be given to events before 1965 in achieving lower fertility, and promoting early knowledge about family planning and safe motherhood.[22] Without the repatriation of Indian Tamils from the 1960s onwards, and the

---

[19]Ibid. pp. 744–746.

[20]For a male to be eligible for a vasectomy, he had to be under the age of 50, and a woman undergoing tubal ligation had to be younger than 45 years on the date of surgery. They had to be a legally married couple, with at least two living children on the date of sterilization. Consent was assured through the implementation of a counseling support system and extensive evaluation, including interviews with female acceptors who were generally grateful for the government services. Wright, N. H, 2007, op. cit. p. 356.

[21]Yapa, L. & Siddhisena, P, 1998, op. cit. p 179.

[22]ibid

outflow of Tamils escaping political violence in the 1980s, the population may have been significantly higher.[23]

Arising from my time in Bangladesh, where I developed some awareness of the importance of data (in part, because of the pioneering work of the Cholera Research Laboratory in Matlab Thana),[24] I was surprised to find that when I arrived, the early eighties, the most popular methods of fertility control in Sri Lanka, unlike later, were sterilization and the use of traditional methods. To my mind, tradition on the one hand and a progressive approach to equal rights on the other, should have suggested otherwise. Interestingly, not only was sterilization the most common form of contraception across the entire country in all regions, the highest rates occurred in the plantation sector of Badulla and the irrigation settlements in the districts of Ampara, Polonnaruwa, and Anuradhapura. All were our project target areas. Regarding the rhythm method, I was told it was popular with conservative Sri Lankan society, a strata who were apprehensive about other birth control measures. Irrespective of literacy and urbanisation, the cultural practice was abstinence after birth, even after ovulation resumed. In the early eighties, twice as many more women were opting for traditional practices than modern temporary methods such as the pill or condoms.[25] I wondered why. At the time my colleagues speculated that the poor diffusion of modern methods was because people were fearful about the programme. But why? The historical promotion of traditional methods, an overly medical approach to the subject of family planning, and poor field work performance, was the response.[26] No one mentioned ethnic tensions as a reason. After 1980, the national effort moved forward decisively, and it was the sterilization programme that was ultimately effective in helping complete Sri Lanka's demographic transition.[27]

As I digested this information, I was conscious that my counterparts instinctively knew what the issues were and how best to direct the Ministry's efforts. They were constantly in touch with their provincial colleagues and, through them, the nominated target audiences. For me to make my contribution it was now time to get settled.

Not long after we arrived and moved into our residence in Pepin Lane, I was sitting in a local Chinese Restaurant having my lunch. I was reading

---

[23]Wright, N. H. 2007, op. cit. 358.

[24]Matlab, a rural area, about 50 km south of Dhaka is one of the richest and longest running longitudinal data source of developing world.

[25]Wright, N.H. 2007, op cit. p. 184.

[26]Unfortunately, while no direct data supports the incidents of induced abortion, cases relating to complications from induced abortions rose 30% between 1970–1985, and was no doubt linked to the pressure to have smaller families.

[27]Wright, N. H. 2007, op. cit. p. 357–359.

the latest edition of the Manchester Guardian (another icon like the BBC that has sustained me through all my postings), when it dawned on me that I had only been in Sri Lanka for four weeks and I was already behaving like a local, at ease in my surroundings.[28] Did it reflect my adaptability, lessons learnt from previous transitions or had it more to do with the welcome given by the Sri Lankans and the cultural linkages they shared with an expatriate Australian? Maybe it was the Buddhist tradition or my welcomed relief at being able to move freely in a society far less restrained by any sexual divide? Given that I have often struggled in the first six months of a new assignment, I suspect it was both. After Bangladesh, Sri Lanka was a welcome interlude. Because the country was sufficiently small to enable a total view and sufficiently varied, I was never bored. In a matter of miles you could move from tropical vegetation, to dry scrub, to 7000-foot plateaus with spectacular views and then down to glorious coastlines. You could visit ancient Buddhist ruins of grandeur, chase the peacocks with my daughter around the garden at our sports club or sit in front of a roaring fire in a house built for a Scottish tea planter sharing a devonshire tea. Home at night in Pepin Lane with the air-conditioners on and the ceiling fans whirling, saw us all watching television together, the nanny, the cook, the daughter, the niece, and myself.

My new office was in the stand-alone Ministry of Labour building where all the departmental staff were located. One of the staff from the driver's pool was allocated to me as my driver. His contribution formed part of the government's contribution to the projects for which I was responsible. Each morning he would collect me having driven backwards down our narrow lane. There was no room to turn around so the traffic would wait on that busy main road while he performed this manoeuvre. He was an irascible character whose typical work attire was a shirt worn outside his sarong and a pair of flip-flops. My counterparts being senior labour officials, had spent their entire careers in the bureaucracy beginning as rural labour commissioners before being transferred to the headquarters. They knew everyone. Before long so did I. I was made very welcome. It was a camaraderie among men (and they were all men) with shared experiences. They were competent project administrators who knew all the ILO players in Bangkok and Geneva and had the ILO's development treadmill well sussed out. They were in the "know" and well-versed in its arts. Included in their numbers were colleagues who would later follow each other into the international bureaucracy. I was still an amateur, and although keen to push forward, culturally limited in my ability to play the game.

---

[28]Letters to parents, 2 May, 1980.

During my time in Sri Lanka I was basically a bureaucrat. I wrote ministerial speeches, drafted departmental position papers, and made submissions to the planning ministry. As I read the files, developed a network of contacts and listened to my colleagues, I began to think about how best to formulate a national strategy and then translate it into a programme for training plantation and industrial workers to deliver health services. I queried whether our training efforts, admirable as they were, were just one-off exercises run according to an annual target of activities required to be completed? Were those essential linkages there between the education given and the service delivery demanded? To answer these questions I sought to gauge how supportive management and the various union federations actually were. Was it lip service they were paying to a cause which, while admirable in intent, was not guaranteed to win them any votes when next they stood for election? Were they prepared to commit resources to funding clinics, financing trained staff, paying for medical supplies, allowing paid time off for workers to be trained and then to attend information sessions? I began to visit each of the various headquarters and question their commitment. Similarly, a round of field trips to the provinces was scheduled where we could question management, inspect the clinics or the first aid station, talk to the unions,[29] and listen to the workers. Over time we put together a checklist. What did people know about family planning? Where did they receive whatever information they had? Were they practising and, if so, what method? Who was responsible? Was there a first aid box, a cupboard, a room or a designated clinic at the work site? Were any staff trained? Did they have the requisite supply of drugs, stored correctly and regularly restocked? Was reproductive health and family planning operationalised and effectively managed? Could at-risk clients be identified and transferred, in time, to a hospital? Did they have a record-keeping system? How were workers being kept informed of what they needed, and did they understand the requirements? It was all very random and rudimentary. So many questions being asked and how I must have irritated them, pushing and probing, writing down answers and trying to piece

---

[29]I began by meeting younger staff of the Ceylon Workers Congress (CWC) who I had met earlier in New Delhi at a International Confederation of Free Trade Unions (ICFTU) training programme. The ICFTU was an international trade union confederation one of whose 225 affiliated organisations in 148 countries and territories was the Fiji Trade Union Congress with whom I was employed prior to joining the ILO. The ICFTU came into being on 7 December 1949 following a split within the World Federation of Trade Unions (WFTU), and was dissolved on 31 October 2006 when it merged with the World Confederation of Labour (WCL) to form the International Trade Union Confederation (ITUC)). My contacts in the CWC introduced me to Savumiamoorthy Thondaman, the legendary union leader and politician who represented the Indian Tamils of Sri Lanka of which he was a member. The CWC had traditionally represented Tamils working in the plantation sector of the economy where appointments seemed to be passed from father to son, evidence the current leadership of the CWC by the grandson of Savumiamoorthy, Arumugam Thondaman.

together whether or not there was an integrated programme and if not, what to do about it. But it was all taken in good spirit. No one ever seemed to mind my impertinence. People seemed genuinely committed to trying to improve the lives of thousands of workers.

All this questioning meant we had to be on site, to see what was actually happening. It was not only a Colombo-based exercise. Extensive travel out of Colombo with my counterparts was required.[30] Together we would head-up-country to the coffee and tea estates or motor down to the coastal plantations of rubber and copra. We travelled to the northern city of Jaffna, Trincomalee in the Eastern Province, many times to Kandy in the Central Province and to the fishing districts of Negombo, Galle Batticaloa, Trincomalee and Kilinochchi. The resident Assistant Commissioner of Labour always hosted us. Typically, this meant that at the end of the day there would be the customary drinking of arak followed by the standard meal of *string hoppers* (i.e. rice flour pressed into a form of noodles and then steamed), hot curry (e.g. potato, egg, fish or meat) and coconut chutney or if we were on the coast, barbecued fish on the beach and more drinking of arak. Then, at nightfall, we joined in singing American and Irish standards, chief among them being the country music songs of Jim Reeve.[31] Inspections to the factories in Colombo or the free-trade zones near the airport were, however, more business-like.

Our main focus were the plantations. Nearly all of them relied on a vast workforce of semi-educated labourers who picked, plucked, smoked, tapped, or dried the crops.[32] They lived with their wives, large numbers of children and their extended families in lines of huts provided by the employer. Jobs were passed on from generation to generation. Many of the estates were previously colonial enterprises run by a resident expatriate manager. Now, all were localised, but the remnants of the colonial lifestyle lingered on in the clubs, the golf links and the traditional observances like a game of billiards and a whiskey after dinner.

---

[30]Letters to parents, 11 September, 1980.

[31]As I discovered throughout my postings if you could happily join in singing karaoke or felt comfortable gathered around a guitar, such inclusions were a universal lingua franca that overcame most cultural differences.

[32]Letters to parents, 21 December 1979.

Soon Colombo was familiar territory. We had settled into a routine. At the ministry I had begun to turn my attention to what needed to be done to move the programme to the next level. After the travel, the reading, and the listening, it was time to begin mapping out an agenda for the departmental secretary to consider. How could the management and the unions do more? Where were the services said to be provided by the concerned ministries? What needed to be done to improve the lives of these workers and their families? Momentum was starting to build. We needed a plan of action. We began to draft a new UNFPA country programme.

But then it was all over. My time was prematurely cut short when the first of many financial crises hit UNFPA following the election of President Reagan in 1981. It began with a steady withdrawal of US funding and culminated in the Global Gag Rule announced at the International Conference on Population held in Mexico City in 1984. UNFPA's budget was slashed. The ILO staff in the Geneva and Bangkok offices who were funded by UNFPA were confronted with reduced funding and had to decide on what needed to be cut and what should be saved. It was the field-based contracted staff who were most vulnerable. That included me. Because Sri Lanka was not a priority country for financial assistance, the proposed new country programme with the government into which all our efforts were being directed, saw the projected budget cut. The expected ministerial approval of the extension to my contract was null and void. My counterparts and I were flailing around trying to redeem something of our projects. Very kindly, the Ministry undertook to use their own funds so I could be temporarily extended while I navigated the approval mechanism for our much-reduced projects while at the same time looked elsewhere for a new assignment. Welcome to the world of consultants! As I had learnt in Bangladesh, one of the challenges of being a contracted United Nations official was that you depended on others for the renewal of your contract as well as the availability of the necessary finance.[33] Putting the two together, in a timely way, was a never-ending challenge, one bound to cause the international expert sleepless nights. I was now in this very position. In the search for a new posting, I was advised to contact all my "friends" in New York, Bangkok and Geneva. I sent off countless letters. Despite supportive replies there was nothing.

At the time, I never questioned the ILO's non-extension of contracts held by myself and other field-based colleagues. I had always welcomed Bangkok and Geneva's support. But soon I realised that while all the service delivery advisor posts were cut, those regionally based staff suffered no staffing cuts.

---

[33]Letters to parents, September 9, 1980.

Nor were there any reductions in Geneva. Even though we were all funded by UNFPA, these bureaucrats looked after themselves while the so-called agents of change at the front-line, those who provided the primary rationale for the funding, were let go. Years later at times of comparable crises, I resolved that it was the field-based staff the UN needed to retain, not those at the headquarters or in the regional offices. Now, in those early years of my UN career when I was trying to shape a future for myself, I became caught between my very limited UN experience and no experience at all back at in Australia. When it came to seeking favours I was reluctant to do so, culturally presuming inclusiveness and the assumption that my colleagues would tell me if any jobs were available. But ILO assistance was not just about the transformative effectiveness of development aid. It was about keeping your post in the comfortable surrounds of a UN office block. During a time of budget cuts, loyalty to far distant staff only went so far. Because I was on a project that had a limited life, I was always subject to the availability of finance, the approval of my counterparts and the satisfactory performance reports from my supervisor in Bangkok. That was and remains the reality of a consultant's life. When the project ends, you wonder if there will be another assignment and, if so, where it will be. You apply, you wait, months pass without hearing anything. Then, should there be a positive response, you are expected to be ready within the week. In the interim, out of necessity you have moved on with your life, so much so that when the offer comes, you hesitate because now, as was often the case, there is just not you but your partner and the future of your children to consider, notably their education. Do you want them to be with you, enrolled at a local international school or do you prefer to enrol them in boarding school back home, which, in my case, was Australia (or anywhere for that matter)? And what of the "accompanying spouse"? They have their personal goals, career ambitions and family and cultural needs. Often, they are torn between wanting to be with their partner and alienation from their surroundings, made critically so when they are denied local work permits. In Colombo in the early eighties I struggled with these conflicting emotions. Perhaps it would be best if I returned to be closer to my ageing parents and extended family. But what would I do? It would mean starting again, looking for a job. That was not going to be easy. No longer would I be an aspiring ILO adviser keen to carve out a career in the UN family of development workers. Gone would be that commitment and with it the status of working for the United Nations. There would be no future in that dream or so it seemed. Without a contract, unemployment beckoned.[34] In the short time remaining

---

[34]Letters to parents, 12 July 1980.

the ILO instructed me to go on leave and use up all my entitlements. The Maldives beckoned.

The flight to Mali, the capital of the Maldives, did not mean had reached its destination. If you had a booking at one of the far-flung islands, you took a boat from the airport to whatever of the islands was your chosen venue. No doubt it is still the same. Like all the other islands, ours was small and on a coral atoll. I quickly discovered we could walk around it in 20 min. Overwhelmingly, the resort catered to the sophisticated European or so it seemed to my jaundiced eye. The female guests would come to breakfast in their high heels with their sarong discreetly covering their bikini. Husbands wore their Bermuda shorts and carried thick volumes to be read over breakfast while their wives stared into the distance. We quickly discovered that any eye contact with the other guests let alone a cheery Aussie greeting created some consternation breaking as it was the discreet eating of your pawpaw. We learnt not to invade the territory of the neighbouring tables. I remember it as all very controlled and in a letter to my parents said it reminded me of Jacques Tati's famous film, "Monsieur Hulot's holiday". Still, we were relaxed. And so, it would have continued, had it not been for the arrival on the horizon of the USS Enterprise, the world's first nuclear-powered aircraft carrier and the eighth United States naval vessel to bear the name. There it stood one early morning, this gigantic monster, at 342 m the longest naval ship in the world. Fresh from patrolling the vastness of the Indian Ocean, its crew were now on R&R. Soon they were pouring ashore from their amphibious landing craft. With their 'master blasters'[35] blaring, I expected our European sophisticates to turn their noses away with disdain. They didn't. Instead, they enthusiastically responded to the invitation to jive a little, drink a little and why not wander down the beach so I could get to know you better, a little. Suddenly, the whole place was jumping with couples heading off into the undergrowth. I was astonished. I was even more astonished when I heard how the 4,600 crew of the ship had dispersed themselves throughout the Maldives chain, and how the US Navy managed discipline and racial tensions aboard the aircraft carrier. I was told that fines were the main means for correcting bad behaviour. Later, in the afternoon, the various couples began to drift back into the hotel. With the landing craft set to return to the big ship, they embraced, looked longingly into each other's eyes, kissed and then the sailors were gone. The Enterprise disappeared over the horizon. There one minute,

---

[35] "Master Blaster (Jammin)" was a 1980 single by American singer-songwriter Stevie Wonder from his 1980 album Hotter than July. Over time it became a common slang term for a music playing recording machine.

gone the next. I wondered if I'd had a dream. What was not a dream on return to Colombo was the packing up, the farewells and then the flight home. It was all over. It was repatriation to Australia—unemployment and winter. No choice but to start again. Still, I had the memories and a nice letter from Geneva wishing me well.

5

From East to West: Kenya

*"If you think you are too small to make a difference, you haven't spent a
night with a mosquito" African proverb*

"It will only be for a year," I said, referring to a new ILO offer but secretly
hoping it would be extended.[1] It was 1988 and there was no guarantee of
a longer contract but I needed to persuade my wife and children to leave
a stable situation and journey, yet again, to another strange and unknown
continent. After years spent at the development front line, the option of
nesting in our own Australian home was now welcomed by the family. But
once the international lifestyle has a claim on you, it's hard to let go. Commitment to a worthy cause, making a difference, learning by doing, exposure to
the new and the sense that I was good at it and recognised for being so,
propelled me back into the UN system.[2] I wanted to be on that international flight. Selfish, I know, but I was convincing when I said a new UN

---

[1] Recall that owing to the USA funding cuts to UNFPA as a result of the election of the Republicans
and their hostility to the UN, generally, and UNFPA, specifically, I had had a break in service
between the end of my Sri Lankan assignment and my appointment to Kenya. Another feature of
the eighties, which continues today, is that the global aid project increasingly focused away from Asia
to Africa. This meant that when countries in South East Asia reached middle income status foreign
aid was often withdrawn and redirected to Africa.

[2] Not that everyone saw it this way. When we told people we were going to Africa, many were
not only taken aback, they said that once there you'll get every disease known to humanity. Plus
there's tribalism, internal warfare, and every possible calamity! For the first time I saw how people
had such biased or rather uninformed views about Africa. There are so many misconceptions. Even

---

© The Author(s), under exclusive license to Springer Nature
Switzerland AG 2021
I. Howie, *Reflections on a United Nations' Career*, Springer Biographies,
https://doi.org/10.1007/978-3-030-77063-1_5

appointment would be in the interests of all of us. My wife reluctantly agreed but determined that I would have to go ahead with her and the children to follow. They would await the end of the first school term plus the ILO's authorisation of payment for transporting our air freight from Australia to Kenya.

It was the musical score to the film "Out of Africa", starring Robert Redford and Meryl Streep, that I was recalling when I had my pre-travel injections in Melbourne. Medical friends had warned me that Africa was rife with health challenges. "Be prepared!" they said. It will be worth it, I thought, as I was immunised against every disease imaginable. That said, I was soon airborne on the long flight north to ILO Headquarters in Geneva.

Unlike my first visit twelve years earlier, I now felt like an old hand in this diplomatic enclave. I stayed at the Windsor Hotel in the centre of the city and even asked the office to book it for me. I was on familiar terms with the hotel staff, who were still decked out in jacket and tie and I relished the morning breakfast of crisply baked rolls and fresh jam. I even felt part of the daily crowd as they waited at the bus station. Once at the ILO, I no longer dashed from office to office. Briefing was now as anticipated. Perfectly natural then was the flight from Geneva to Nairobi where, on arrival, I knew what awaited me: the need to find a house, set up an office, recruit staff, be introduced to counterparts, and, once settled, plan the way forward to make that "difference".

The title of my post in Kenya,[3] and the accompanying job description, were generic and could be applied anywhere throughout the world. I was charged with introducing a workers' family welfare education and services programme in the 'organised sector' (i.e. in 100 large industries via the management, the trade unions and the peak employer bodies). In the words of the project document, the primary objective was to develop and pilot an "operations model" for integrating family welfare programmes via the Ministry of Labour into the ongoing operations of plantations and facto-ries.[4] Also included was a second but minor project targeted specifically at women and youth in the slum areas of Nairobi. Here I was expected to pilot a scheme for NGOs bringing maternal and child health along with family

---

today, many think Africa is one country or when you talk about the continent, they can only think of South Africa.

[3]"Expert in Labour, Population/Family Welfare Education" job description.

[4]The plantation sector consisted of tea estates centred around the township of Kericho, the sizel estates located along the coast and the coffee farms scattered throughout the high country of Kenya. The factories were varied and included car assembly, pharmaceuticals, concrete, tourism, and ports.

planning to their outreach programmes. How to meet both these goals was up to me as had been the case in Bangladesh and Sri Lanka. Still, the overall responsibilities were clear. Decide and then test, through trial and error, how best to improve the health outcomes of workers employed in these industries, especially those outcomes associated with birth spacing and safe motherhood. In addition to the management and the unions, the other possible entry points were the clinics, or first aid stations located within the firms and those staff, if there were any, charged with looking after the health of the workers and their families. Their contact with the ministries of health, labour, rural development, and agriculture would be important. Equally important would be training my counterparts in the Ministry to take responsibility for the project after I left. These then were the parameters, but because it was a pilot project, I was again starting from scratch. I did have, however, the project delivery model I had road tested in Bangladesh and Sri Lanka. What I needed to do now was adjust that experience and apply it to the Kenyan situation. But what was that situation? To help me answer that question, the ILO in Geneva had given me a description of the country, an outline of the broad population and health parameters, a paragraph or two on the institutional base where I was to be located and a description of my counterparts whom I would meet when I arrived (all, a marked improvement from my earlier experiences). To that I added my rudimentary knowledge of East Africa. Included here was my vague recollection that some of the earliest fossilized remains of hominids dating back millions of years had been discovered in Kenya. I also recalled hearing Tom Mboya, the trade unionist and one of the founding fathers of the Republic of Kenya, speak in Melbourne in 1964 when I was a student. Like others, I was mightily impressed with his eloquence and passion. I had read the novel "White Mischief" by James Fox, a fictionalized account of the unsolved murder in 1941 of Josslyn Hay, the Earl of Erroll, a British expatriate in Kenya (as well as seen the 1987 film adaption). I knew of the books of Karen Blixen, the Danish author best known for her book "Out of Africa", an account of her life while living in Kenya. Clearly, my knowledge was totally inadequate. I had a lot more learning to do. To begin, I needed to know something about the history of Kenya including what efforts had been made, if any, to improve the "family life" of workers.

What struck me from my initial reading about Kenya was that it was both a vibrant country, with a colourful past, as well as a country of balance. Being located between the Great Rift Valley[5] and the banks of Lake Victoria, it was culturally diverse with its population mix of traditional tribes and urban families, of ancient traditions and modern challenges. The tourist, typically focused on safaris to the big game parks or the beaches on the Swahili Coast, often missed the centuries old pre-colonisation trading relations between southern Arabia and the coastline whose evidence in Mombasa and the island of Lamu,[6] so delighted me. Tourists rarely ventured to the thriving townships on the Lake or to the plantation areas in the Valley. They also knew little of the contemporary history whereby, what is known today as Kenya and Uganda were, until 1920, part of the British East Africa Protectorate. As I was reminded when posted to Rwanda, the Berlin Conference of 1885 saw East Africa divided into territories by the European powers (Germany, Britain, and France). Three years later in 1888 with Britain and Germany both competing for control of the coast and its hinterland, the British East African Company was granted a charter to open up the highlands and the fertile valley to white settlers, displacing the African tribes like the Masai and Kikuyu.[7] European migration increased thereafter until the start of the 1914–18 war. Many Asians had already settled, being first recruited as labourers on the construction of the railway linking the port of Mombasa with Kisumu on Lake Victoria, 1895–1901. With Nairobi now the headquarters of the British administration and these white settlers having a voice in government, it was only in 1944 that African and Asians were no longer banned from direct political participation. In that year the Kenyan African Union (KAU) was formed to campaign for independence. In 1947 Jomo Kenyatta became the leader of KAU. He had spent most of the 1930s and 40 s campaigning in Europe for African territorial economic and political rights. Then in 1952 a secret Kikuyu guerrilla group known as the Mau Mau[8] began a violent campaign against white settlers. A state of emergency was declared. It continued for the next 8 years. The struggle for independence had begun.

---

[5]The Great Rift Valley is a geographical and geological feature running north to south for around 4,000 miles (6,400 km), from northern Syria to central Mozambique in East Africa (http://www.new worldencyclopedia.org/entry/Great_Rift_Valley).

[6]When the Portuguese arrived in 1498, the Arab dominated coast because an important resupply stop for ships bound for the Far East. In the late 1600s the Portuguese gave way and the coast came under Islamic control by the Imam of Oman.

[7]Kenya comprises 47 different tribes: 67% Buntu (Kikuyu, Luhya, Kamba), 30% Nilotic (Kalenjin, Luo), 3% other (Cushitic, Arabs, Indians, Europeans). The Kikuya are the largest ethnic group in Kenya.

[8]The Mau Mau were a militant African nationalist movement among the Kikuyu people of Kenya. The Mau Mau advocated violent resistance to British domination in Kenya.

During this time Kenyatta was arrested and jailed (1953–61), the KAU was banned (1953) and the Mau Mau rebellion put down by a combination of British military operations. In 1960 the Kenya African National Union (KANU) was formed by Tom Mboya and Oginga Odinga (a distinguished Luo as was Mboya). Once freed from jail, Kenyatta resumed the presidency becoming the nation's first president in 1964 following independence from the British in December 1963.[9] He remained so until his death in 1978. Jomo Kenyatta is often referred to as Kenya's founding father, rightly seen as a great African statesman—proof of the clichéd truism that *"one man's terrorist is another's freedom fighter"*, and that gaining power is the best form of rehabilitation.[10] After Kenyatta's death, Daniel arap Moi[11] succeeded him. Initially, the transition from such a dominant figure took place smoothly with Moi following Kenyatta's policy of distributing offices among as many different ethnic groups as possible. But in 1982 he declared that KANU was to be the sole legal party. With that curtailing of democracy, foreign aid was suspended. It wasn't until late 1991 that Moi bowed to domestic and foreign pressure and agreed to accept a multi-party-political system. Despite the opposition parties' best efforts, they failed to dislodge KANU in the 1992 and 1997 elections and Moi remained in power until 2002.[12] During that time he had seen to it that members of his own Kalenjin group had acquired a disproportionate number of appointments.[13] After 24 years in power and now bound by the constitution which limited presidential office to two terms, Moi was finally forced to stand down. He was succeeded by Uhuru Kenyatta, Jomo Kenyatta's son who in October 2017 was re-elected for a second term. Despite the political upheavals and calamitous elections, the country has experienced, Kenya today remains the financial hub for both East and Central Africa. It has the highest GDP in the region. In 1988 when I arrived, it was said by UN colleagues to be "… a dream compared to the rest of Africa."[14]

When I reached Nairobi, it was raining. Indeed, it was the rainy season throughout the country. Although not the monsoon time, it did rain a lot. Fortunately, it seemed to do so at night. During the day it was cloudy but not that hot (low to mid twenties). Greyness seemed to characterise my early

[9] http://www.bbc.com/news/world-africa-13682176.

[10] John Andrews, *"The World in Conflict"*, The Economist, London, 2015.

[11] Moi came from Sacho, a small tribe located on the edge of Lake Victoria in Western Kenya. He was initially seen as an interim President.

[12] Andrews op cit, pxx.

[13] Paul Nugent, AFRICA SINCE INDEPENDENCE, Second Edition (Palgrave Macmillan, Basingstoke, 2012), pp 418–422.

[14] Letter to parents, July 1st, 1998.

days. The weeks that followed were, in retrospect, not particularly demanding or stressful. By now I knew something of the realities of living in a developing country. Kenya, being a former British colony, meant they spoke English and drove on the "correct" side of the road. I stayed initially at the United Kenya Club. I chose the Club because it was not far from the government building where my office was. They offered me a room with attached shower plus two meals a day. There was a billiard room, a reading room and a lounge with an attached bar. All fairly basic but adequate and reasonable. Being new, I was a stranger in a strange land. There was no hint of any invitations from either my new workmates at the ministry or the UN. With no family or social life, I often lay on my bed at night reading books.[15] One day I plucked up courage and introduced myself to others sitting silently by themselves across the dining room. I worked on remembering their names and suggested we explore Nairobi together. All enthusiastically agreed and we set out. Endless walks ensued as we found our bearings. I also quizzed my new friends about life in Nairobi. Did they know how I might find a place for the family to live and where should I buy furniture, curtains, stoves and fridges et cetera?[16] I had been scanning newspapers and reading notice boards. It was like piecing together a jigsaw puzzle and while challenging I was told repeatedly how easy it was here in Kenya compared with other African countries. I usually remembered this as I walked from office to office queueing for yet another form to be signed! Still, from this small gesture of reaching out to others in that dining room I learnt something about how to combat loneliness, a reality with which consultants on short term assignments often struggle. But for me this all changed when I was contacted by a Gudgerati family whose relatives I had known in Fiji inviting me to stay.

In pursuit of accomodation for my soon to arrive family I discovered that opposite my office building was a large block of apartments. Known as "Bishops Gardens" it was owned by the Anglican Church. In its spacious grounds there was parking, a swimming pool, flowering jacaranda trees,

---

[15]Over time, when travelling by myself I came to rely more and more on access to a gym, reading the Guardian newspaper and listening to the World Service of the BBC. These were the ever-present accoutrements to my international life.

[16]Important to note here is that the UN is not like the Australian diplomatic corps where most things are provided to the newly arrived diplomat (including furnished accommodation). As noted earlier, the UN official has to learn his or her way around as best they can. This means finding a house and figuring out where to buy all the things your new house needs including determining what is a fair price, often in countries where bargaining is the norm, and where brand names mean nothing to you. And, all this in a currency with which you are not familiar. Then there are the government requirements for visas, work permits, driver's licenses, official photos, identity cards, opening bank accounts, registering for duty-free entitlements etc.—all, via a bureaucracy which is notoriously slow and cumbersome.

oleanders, and an expanse of lawn where children could play. It was well guarded by *ascaris* (Swahili term for night watchmen) at the main gate. Further enquiries revealed there was a vacant two-storied, four bedroom flat on the ground floor. I tracked down the agent and did a deal. It would be available when the family arrived. What a relief as comfort and security for the family were an absolute priority.

Later, when we moved in, we were again reminded that one of the joys of an international life are the friends you make. At "Bishop's Gardens" they came from all corners of the globe. Next door was a Finnish couple with three daughters. Further down and upstairs were Norwegians, Portuguese, Swedes, Danes, Tanzanians, Americans and even a number of the old Africa hands, originally from the UK, but now after one or two generations part of the post-colonial landscape. On the down side, was the constant departure of families whom you befriended on arrival only to see them transferred to another country as they came to the end of their assignments (a reality all expatriates face and which came to us soon enough). Living a transient life means welcomes today and farewells tomorrow.[17]

Another adjustment was the government prohibition preventing married partners from obtaining work permits. As a UN adviser I had a permit. My wife did not.[18] For any professional women wanting to pursue their skills and careers this was unjust. In our case, the demands of a new city, a new house, a new baby and new schooling for an older child meant there was a full-time occupation for my 'accompanying spouse'. Later, once settled but with no employment possible, my wife trained as a volunteer guide with the Kenya Museum, an activity she thoroughly enjoyed.

In keeping with standard UN practice there was the executing agency to which I belonged (i.e. the ILO) and a funding agency (i.e. UNFPA). There was also the local implementing agency which in Kenya, as was the case in Sri Lanka, was the Department of Labour. In overall charge of the project was a departmental deputy secretary. Officially, he was the project director. Unofficially, it was pointed out to me that he came from the largest ethnic group in Kenya, the Kikuyus. Apart from being a tribal designation this meant little to me at the time. When I met him, he immediately asked that I write a speech for the Minister for Manpower Development. It was to be delivered, the director told me, at a seminar my counterparts and I were to arrange

---

[17]Equally draining were the emotional farewells with our parents, following home leave, when we headed off back to Nairobi from Melbourne. You pay a cost living away from home and family. At that time, home leave for international project staff in the UN system in Kenya was applicable once every two years, provided your contract had more than six months to go before expiring.

[18]Kenya was not alone in this respect; it was common practice in many developing countries.

for late July in Nyeri located in the Kenyan Highlands. This was to be a National Orientation Seminar for the umbrella organisations, COTU and FKE. We needed their support and their approval to approach local union leaders (to allay any fears that our programme was a management ploy not in the best interests of union members), and to approach management (to either enter a factory premise and/or to allow the distribution of contraceptives). In preparation, my early research told me that the Kenyan workforce stood at 7.5 million in 1985 and was expected to grow to 14 million by 2000. Given the modest economic growth rate forecast, this suggested that Kenyan parents were having more children than they could care for. Further reading revealed that fertility and population growth in Kenya—reputed to be the highest in the world—may have been dropping, according to the preliminary results of a Kenyan Demographic and Health Survey (KDHS). The KDHS, Kenya's third such survey on fertility, family planning, and maternal/child health, reported that the nation's total fertility rate (TFR) was 6.7.[19] This stood in contrast to the 7.7 figure reported by a similar survey in 1984. It was also a significant decline from 1980 to 1985, when, according to the World Population Prospects 1988 (UN Department of International and Social Affairs, 1989), the TFR was 8.1. This recent decline in fertility, said the KDHS, was consistent with increases in contraceptive use. A total of 27% of all married women were now found to be using some form of contraception (two-thirds of which were common methods)—a 50% increase since the 1984 survey. The KDHS reported only minor urban-rural differentials in the level of contraceptive use, which suggested that services and supplies were reaching the countryside.[20]/[21] My speech for the minister concluded by declaring that our project was going to be a challenging one but anticipated were further changes in fertility behaviour.

There were two counterparts. When I first arrived to meet them, they were formally dressed in suits and ties. Language was also formal. The taller of the two was a thin man who proudly said he was a Lua from the Lake Victoria region. I was learning that one's tribe mattered. The other was a shorter,

---

[19]The TFR is the entire number of births a woman would have if she passed through her childbearing years conforming to current age-specific fertility rates.

[20]"Kenya's fertility: no longer the world's highest?" POPULATION UNFPA NEWSLETTER, VOL. 15 NO 11 p.2. That said, in 2019, 1 million were being added to the Kenyan population each year. https://www.worldbank.org/en/news/opinion/2010/04/28/demographic-transition-growth-kenya.

[21]Of more concern should have been the high rates of maternal mortality which even today have not markedly improved. 2019 data shows that 342 women die per 100,000 live births in Kenya with adolescent girls at a higher risk of death as a result of pregnancy. A chronic absence of staff exacerbates the situation. Devex "Access to Contraception" in 3 multimedia stories: A Closer look at Kenya's maternal care". 5 December 2019.

chain-smoking man who told me he came from the same tribe as the President, the Kisii people from the Rift Valley region. Over time, I saw that there was no great love lost between the two. Nor did they ever seek to be more than work colleagues to me. There was never any contact beyond the office nor any suggestion that there might be. But we collaborated well enough. They were my counterparts, after all, with whom I needed to interact and train, and whose briefings would help me undertake the work with which I was charged.

Apart from meeting my new colleagues in that first week, I also needed to prepare an office for myself and any staff I would employ. When it came to supplies I was told "It's all in the basement. Why don't you go down there and pick up whatever you need". I headed downstairs but after greeting the officer-in-charge, I was told there were no stores. The department had no money, he said. What about the commitment made in the project document to provide those basic items? He had no idea what I was talking about. But don't be disappointed, he roared with a laugh, no-one in the government had any money! I came away empty-handed. Instead of these supplies being covered by counterpart funding, I would have to use project budgets to buy them. I searched for a shop where I could buy pens, drawing pins, sticky tape, staplers, rubber bands and typewriter ribbon etc. They weren't difficult to find. There were many outlets and the concerned supplier did well out of our projects, providing letterhead stationery, business cards and all the paraphernalia that any functioning office needed in those pre-computerised days. The heavier office furniture we also bought locally.

Under the project budget I was also allocated an amount to employ a secretary. I advertised. I found Grace. She was a Kikuyu but, more telling from my perspective, a single mother and a born-again Christian. Loyal and hard-working, I remember her with great fondness not least because her every sentence ended with "praise the lord". So much so that when I met with the leaders of the Central Organisation of Trade Unions (COTU), the Federation of Kenya Employers (FKE) and the National Council for Population and Development, they all commented, favourably, on her religiosity. When I left Kenya, I secured a permanent appointment for Grace with the UN Environment Programme (UNEP)[22] whose headquarters were on the outskirts of Nairobi. She was set for the rest of her working life.

---

[22]At that time, there were only two UN organisations that had their global HQs in a developing country, and both were in Kenya—UNEP and UN HABITAT. Both were located on the outskirts of Nairobi in the suburb of Gigiri.

In those early days I would walk to the office. I did so because I never knew what time the ministry car allocated to me would turn up or whether it would turn up at all. Although it wasn't far, most locals advised against walking because of the lack of security. "Avoid anything but the most public of places and don't go out at night," they would warn me. In such an environment, the security industry boomed. While I continued to walk everywhere, this flirting with potential danger was solved, in part, when I bought the two Land Rovers allocated under the projects. We needed them to travel outside the capital. In keeping with standard practice, I contacted the UN's, Inter-Agency Procurement Services Office (IAPSU). Based in Copenhagen, it was and remains, the procurement market of the United Nations system where, amongst the many services it offers, projects can order equipment. Unfortunately, contrary to the assurances given to me by IAPSU that the vehicles would soon be delivered, there seemed to be an untimely delay between ordering from the supplier, their shipment to the port of Mombasa, rail transport from Mombasa to Nairobi and our taking delivery of them. As I discovered, the explanation lay elsewhere. One Saturday morning my wife and I after shopping at the market in Central Nairobi were walking back to the car we had bought for our personal use. Imagine my astonishment when, as we came to an intersection and stopped at the lights, I saw a brand-new red Land Rover, complete with diplomatic number plates, also stopped and being driven by one of my two counterparts. The car was jam-packed with its roof rack piled high with goods. There were family members squashed into the front and back seats. My colleague saw me, and I saw him. We looked at each other with surprise until the lights changed and he drove off. Under UN regulations, it was strictly forbidden that project vehicles issued with diplomatic number plates be used for private purposes. That was not to say international staff could not request to use a project vehicle for personal use but the protocol dictated that any mileage travelled had to be recorded and paid for. In this case, we had a local driving a diplomatically registered vehicle for which none of the standard requirements had been met. Here was an early crisis for me. Just as I had learned in previous assignments, relationships with counterparts could be problematic not least because using their local contacts they can make life very difficult for the international expert. As my new counterpart would be required to report on me later in the year, if I embarrassed him now by reporting his improper use of a vehicle, that could be a complication I might never recover from. I was a guest in the country, contracted to advise the ministry and the continuation of my contract for a second year depended on my relationship with, among others, this colleague. But he had flouted the rules. If I were to establish some authority as well as carve out some respect, I needed to report him knowing that if I did, I could potentially see him disciplined and myself ostracised. What to do? After struggling with the dilemma over the weekend, I went to see him on the following Monday. Once in his office I talked through the working arrangements, about the rules regarding the use of the vehicle and about the importance of our future collaboration. I then listened to him until finally we agreed to a set of working parameters governing all staff relationships from now on. The proviso was that I would overlook what I had seen on the weekend. Unfortunately, that wasn't the end of it. He had seen my weakness. Sometime later he absconded with the vehicle again. After confronting him, I had to report the matter to the deputy secretary (Project Director). There were no further difficulties. From this experience and those earlier in Bangladesh, I came to appreciate the challenge international advisers faced when collaborating with counterparts. In some ways you could understand how the gap between the local's material circumstances and one's own led to envy and how the opportunity to profit from foreign aid gave rise to engineering any financial advantage. But the funds allocated for our projects came from taxpayers around the world and were given by governments for the improvement of people's lives. As a consequence, my counterparts and I were all accountable. Later, as I discovered, such behaviour was not only confined to poorly paid public servants. Within the UN system itself, there were those who adopted practices which were financially questionable and frankly dishonest. Fortunately, they were few. But, as I discovered in other postings, the behaviour of your predecessor, and their counterparts, did set precedents that could be very challenging for a newcomer. Once rules are bent or broken, the resulting expectations from government officials, irrespective of level, will immediately compromise the effectiveness of the UN official and the integrity of the system itself.

After these opening manoeuvres, it was time I left the capital and visited the locations where our activities were to be operational. We first drove (in the new Land Rover) into Western Kenya reaching as far as Lake Victoria. New towns emerged, at least to me. Kericho, 400 km from Nairobi in the highlands west of the Rift Valley. Here in the hill country were acres and acres of tea planted. It evoked the time I had spent in Darjeeling (India), Nuwara Eliya (Sri Lanka) and Sylhet (Bangladesh). I found the big estates in Kenya were owned by the same companies as was the case in those earlier countries. Brooke Bond, for example, was present although bought out by Unilever in 1984. For me there was something very calming in the orderliness of these high-country estates. They were vast, well-tended, lush, and demarcated by eucalyptus forests and bougainvillea. You looked out across rows and rows of low green bushes rolling over hillsides. In the distance you could pick out the "pluckers" expertly throwing the leaves over their shoulders into the baskets carried on their backs. Like Sri Lanka the workers lived on the estate with their families in "lines" of low-cost but basic housing. The manager always seemed to live elsewhere typically in a bungalow built in earlier times, probably by a Scot. Would that his workers enjoyed the same comforts!

Leaving Kericho it was the road down to Kisumu on the Lake and then back home via Eldoret and Nakuru. Each town had a variety of businesses I was keen to visit. Breweries, textile factories, bakeries, battery manufacturers, sisal estates and sugar plantations. They were among the 100 large firms the project needed to link into. Each employed more than 300 workers. I met management, personnel staff, doctors, nurses, local government officers, adult educators, trade union representatives and workers. I listened as they told me what they did and, importantly, what they would like to do. My task was to determine how best to channel into their workplaces basic government services centred on primary health care, safe motherhood and family planning. I decided to adapt the two-year model I developed in Bangladesh. With my counterparts I drew up a timeline covering contact, registration, needs assessment, factory nominations, training, materials' development, factory IEC, links into the government infrastructure and delivery of services, on-site.

The week-long seminar for union and employer leaders in Nyeri, foreshadowed by the project director at our first meeting, then fell due. Nyeri is a city situated in the densely populated and fertile Central Highlands forming part of the eastern end of the Great Rift Valley. Located about 150 km north of Nairobi, it is one of the oldest towns in Kenya, having been established in the British colonial era. It is also the birthplace of the Boy Scout movement and hosts the tomb of the founder Lord Baden Powell. After the seminar, we travelled down from the valley to the coast where we stayed in the ancient port city of Mombasa, the country's oldest and second-largest city. It has a history of Portuguese, Omani and British occupation and is now a centre of coastal tourism in Kenya. The hotel employees working along the coast were our target audience. But for me Mombasa Island was the main attraction. It is the area I liked best with its narrow streets of the Old Town leading down to Fort Jesus. Built in the late 16th century I stayed in walking distance of the Fort at the wonderful colonial era relic, the Mombasa Club, on the aptly named Sir Mbarak Hinawy Road.

On return from this field trip, I plunged into the slums of Nairobi to initiate the second of my two projects. More new names. The Mathare Valley,[23] Kibera[24] and "Eastlando". Thousands of people living in cramped rusted-roofed shanty towns. All infamous for many things; from insecurity, rampant crime, deplorable public amenities to poor housing and infrastructure. But all alive and thriving. On my first day I walked gingerly through the mud waving to school children, ducking under washing, avoiding the sparks from the open furnaces (*jua-kali*) and greeting the drunks who wanted to engage with this strange visitor. I decided to design a programme working through church-based NGOs that would include education about family life including maternal child health and family planning. This would be located not only among church congregations but also church-supported small-scale enterprises (*jua-kali*). From the start I knew this was going to be a challenge. Fortunately, I met and befriended a social worker employed by the National Council of Churches who became my counterpart. He had links with many NGOs working in the Valley. He was enthusiastic to produce results. Through him I was soon introduced to a multiplicity of youth centres, sports clubs, church congregations and cultural groups. During the next two years we organised the training of 200 women and youth in a number of rudimentary skills related to small-scale industry. This was about bookkeeping, marketing, banking, and credit control. But it also extended to information on population and development. These communities of slum-dwellers never ceased to amaze me with their determination to make the best of their wretched surroundings and their aspirations for a better life, no matter the obstacles. I would visit them every week and as we talked, share a favourite meal of spiced *sukuma wiki* (kale) with meat and *ugali* (cornmeal porridge).

---

[23]The Mathare Valley was one of the oldest and one of the worst slum areas in Nairobi during the nineties. People lived in 6 ft. × 8 ft. shanties made of old tin and mud. There were no beds, no electricity, and no running water. People slept on pieces of cardboard on the dirt floors of the shanties. The public toilets were shared by up to 100 people and residents had to pay to use them. Those who could not afford to pay used the alleys and ditches between the shanties. "Flying toilets" were plastic bags used by the residents at night, then thrown into the Nairobi River, which was the source of the residents' water supply. Today, approximately 600,000 people live in an area of three-square miles. Most live on an income of less than a dollar per day. Crime and HIV/AIDs are common. Many parents die of AIDS and leave their children to fend for themselves. Mathare Community Outreach tries to care for as many of these orphans as possible, but their resources are limited. Source: Wikipedia.

[24]Following the reimposition of the global gag rule by President Trump in 2017, the cuts to IPPF services were such that the outreach FP clinic arrived once a month in Kibera instead of three to four times. Sarah Boseley," 'Global gag' The policy that forces women into deadly procedures" The Guardian Weekly 24 May 2019.

As the months rolled on, I found I was continuously travelling out of the capital to all parts of the country. By now the Ministry had given me a permanent driver. Because I had earlier valued the association I had with the drivers on my projects, this new appointment was one closely anticipated. I would be spending a lot of time with them. They were critical. Contrary to the advice of my counterparts, I managed to persuade the director that a female driver from the ministerial pool would set an affirmative precedent. By good fortune, Janet was assigned. She was a short, strong woman and one well able to hold her own among the league of male drivers.

Meanwhile, my counterparts were very busy organising orientation rallies for thousands of managers and workers to be followed by one week's training of union nominees, usually a shop steward, as our project representatives. This was the model I had deployed earlier in Bangladesh. The nominees came from our target factories and plantations and following the training, were expected to return to their places of work, organise meetings of workers, train and motivate them and then link them up via their factory clinics or estate medical store to the government health services. Typically we would go to a factory/plantation, meet with the management (courtesy of FKE) or, if there was a union, meet with them (courtesy of COTU), and if there was a clinic or first aid shelter and trained health worker meet with them also. The aim was to get a feel for the realities of the working environment, see where the workers lived, how they lived and their circumstances. By these contacts we would piece together a mosaic of the whole infrastructure, starting with the Ministry of Health through to the factories, the plantations and whatever was available or not. Once the groundwork was laid, we would bring in the key people for training, either at a local training centre or in a conference room of a hotel. We would train for a week and include the key local government people from the health department, the labour department and the hospital. We were trying to set up linkages across the departments and break down the silos of local government. By this means, we trained 1,163 participants in 12 months.

To reinforce these networks, we began to follow-up the trainees to ensure that the workforce at their factories or plantations were introduced to the issues. Big rallies were held at which all the key players from management down to the first aid station attendant would speak. It was critical to highlight the key role of the district health centre as a service accessible at the workplace. I had now learnt to stress that training was never an end in itself. It had to consist of action. The challenge was always to consolidate the links between those trained "motivators for change" and the relevant government outreach programmes. Fortunately, following one of our rallies I met the national director of the NGO, Family Planning International Assistance (FPIA) who agreed that, in association with the Ministry of Health, they would supply participating firms with contraceptives, even those that needed a physical examination and a prescription. This was an enormous relief.[25] As an action-based programme involving changes in workers' social behaviour, once a demand was created it had to be regularly serviced. Institutionalisation via the concerned government departments and not our externally funded UN project, was key.

The publicity we received at each of our training venues helped us. Provided we arranged transport and included a free lunch, reporters were happy to cover our events. Using our training budget for this purpose was a reality I came to accept. To be heard on national radio or seen on television, was a big plus for both our participants and the department. As a result of the publicity, I was invited to speak at the May Day celebrations organised by COTU. This was going to be a huge rally in Uhuru Park, Nairobi, and I should have been pleased but I was apprehensive. I recalled my experience in Bangladesh when my counterpart didn't welcome the public accolades accorded to me by government officials. He was the forgotten player or so he felt. The matter was decided though when the programme was printed, and my name appeared as a keynote speaker (one among many). I should not have worried. My counterparts were not there. Nor, I suspect, were they interested in being there. I spoke, receiving a roar of support when I finished.

I now saw the possibility of using the audio-visual resources of our participants far beyond what we could possibly offer them. There were two significant skills to be utilised. One was that in many factories, particularly the clothing and car manufactures, there were art departments, media personnel, advertising staff and marketing people. It occurred to me that for our information, education, communication, and promotional materials, who better to use than these art and advertising departments? We discussed the idea to get them all together and have them design posters that they thought applicable to their circumstances. The management agreed. We had one hundred or so of these very talented people come together at a workshop. We brainstormed, we piloted, and we tested the clarity of the messages and then they returned to their work and set about devoting part of their advertising budget to promoting our issues, be it birth spacing or safe motherhood or contraception. It worked remarkably well. Their designs were printed on

---

[25] Health workers had to venture into the slums just as the district nurses needed to go into the factories.

thousands of *kikoys*[26] and displayed on advertising hoardings throughout the country.

Arising from this success, I then met with the biggest manufacturer of matchboxes, and matches, in the country. I proposed that they put simple messages on every matchbox being manufactured? My thinking was that with most people cooking with charcoal or kerosene or smoking, everyone had a matchbox. Wanted was simple line drawings that promoted good nutrition, breastfeeding, birth spacing, unwanted pregnancies and so on. I explained how these messages could not be complicated nor confusing but instantly understandable. The manufacturer went through with the proposal. They produced millions of matchboxes with our simple line drawings. I was particularly pleased.

Despite the numbers of personnel we trained, this was described in the Kenya Times as a "modest" project given the few project staff involved and the UNFPA financial contribution.[27] However, in terms of an institutionalised package delivering project inputs, no matter how simple and precise they were, it was an ambitious undertaking. That management not only allowed workers time off to be educated but accepted family planning among its staff as its responsibility, was indicative of progress towards the achievement of our long-range objective. That union leaders were also prepared to discuss openly and freely issues presumed to be strictly private and then to publicly accept family planning as a personal responsibility as well as one of concern to their unions, boded well for the future. Finally, that the institutional framework being developed by the Ministry of Labour to establish a contraceptive supply network that would meet the needs of workers suggested we could achieve some future reduction in the population growth rate. But were we achieving these goals? As the months went by, it became increasingly apparent that the motivation of my counterparts in arranging all this training was largely driven by their wanting to save money. Each week away meant the possibility of

---

[26] Kikoys are a traditional wrap-around garment worn on the Swahili coast of East Africa, especially Kenya. It is similar to a sarong and made from hand woven African fabric in the *Jua Kali* industry (outdoor workshops). It is a much more than just a piece of cloth being typically vibrant in colour and symbolising East Africa's culture. It has a hundred different uses and just as many ways to wear it. We also printed on "khangas" which are a similarly colourful garment to a kikoy but worn by women throughout the African Great Lakes region. It is a piece of printed cotton fabric, about 1.5 m by 1 m, often with a border along all four sides, and a central part (*mji*) which differs in design from the borders. One of the longer edges of the *mji* features a strip which contains a message in Swahili, often in the form of riddles or proverbs (from Wikipedia). That is where we printed our family messages message. Unfortunately, a similar idea to include relevant messages in packets of sanitary napkins never advanced beyond the discussion stage with the manufacturer.

[27] Focus on Leaders Population Conference, "Educating the workers", Kenya Times, Wednesday, September 13, 1989.

savings from the travel, accommodation, and daily allowances they received. The rates set by the UN were well above those of the government. They, along with participants, sometimes slept four to a room and with all their meals covered, were able to return home with a welcome amount of cash. I didn't blame them though. Their salaries were meagre. But my concern was that once the project was localised, would they show the same enthusiasm for travel and training? I was doubtful but for the moment, here in Kenya, in the late eighties, we had momentum.[28] As the Kenya Times declared in their headline, we were "Educating the workers".

But then it was all cut short. A pattern was repeated whereby an international advisor associated with projects introducing behavioural change, which take time, moves on. In Bangladesh it was a case of government indifference, in Sri Lanka budget cuts, and now in Kenya my own ambition. I was offered a UNFPA Country Director post in Accra, Ghana, one of 56 such positions around the world (at that time). This offer came on the recommendation of the UNFPA Country Director in Kenya. There was no vacancy announcement but I was asked if I was interested in such as appointment by the officer-in-charge of personnel at UNFPA Headquarters. I was told that I would be the second director posted to Accra and that I would be responsible for a country programme made up of sectoral responsibilities which, in turn, would depend on a set of integrated projects such as those I had been on in Bangladesh, Sri Lanka and Kenya. I would report to the UNDP Resident Representative in Ghana who also held the title of UNFPA Representative.[29] I accepted the offer, although I was concerned where this would leave our Kenyan projects, which were still in their development stage. As mentioned, I doubted the ongoing commitment of my counterparts. Nonetheless, I was assured there would be a new adviser appointed. Besides, I now had the possibility of career development. I was reassured but was concerned how the family would react. It was well past the one-year only promise I gave my wife before we set out for Kenya. Nervously I went home and pitched the argument to her. Carefully, I explained that, in my new capacity, I would represent the Fund and be paid out of the global administrative budget of UNFPA (as distinct from a project post-paid for under a UNFPA Country Programme). Delicately, I added, being against an ongoing 'core post' meant there was now

---

[28]The development concepts I was most attuned to at this time was rooted in the notion of sustainable development. This was an all-embracing concept that had its origin in the 1987 Brundtland Report which, like the earlier basic needs approach, was another initiative of the UN.

[29]Later, the global position of UNFPA Country Director was converted to that of UNFPA Representative with the holders of those positions no longer reporting to the in-country UNDP Resident Representative but to the concerned geographic division director at UNFPA Headquarters.

the opportunity to become a permanent staff member of UNFPA! I would no longer be on a contract attached to a project of set duration. For sweeteners, I added, once in Accra, I would move into an established office within the UN compound. There would even be staff waiting there, already appointed! My wife agreed to this major redirection (I could never have done it without her) and we began planning for our departure including our daughter's future education. That I knew nothing about Ghana nor had ever been there was never a factor in either our or UNFPA's deliberations. I prepared to fly to New York for the orientation.

6

Even Further West: Ghana

Q: *In terms of the work you're doing - as a human being - what keeps you up at night?* A: *Contraceptives. Reproductive health.* Melinda Gates.[1]

Ghana was next in the chain of UN assignments. When we arrived in Accra it was the end of the hottest season. The heat hit us immediately as we began to battle our way through the crowds at the airport while tightly holding onto our children's hands and an assortment of luggage. We did not know what to expect. Would there be someone to meet us? Fortunately, there was. True to form, however, my first six months in Ghana were challenging. I missed Kenya as I would later miss Ghana when I arrived in China. I missed the stunningly beautiful countryside of the Rift Valley and the agreeable climate. I also missed the familiarity of Nairobi—including the Asian family whose members had so welcomed me on arrival in that country. But I wasn't the only one who was challenged at this new posting. Of more concern was the wellbeing of my family.

When initially projected, the peripatetic lifestyle of an international civil servant sounds very attractive. It combines international travel, life in different countries, cultural experiences and meaningful work. But the constant movement can be tough on families. Upheaval, movement and constantly starting again. Add to this, as was the case in Kenya and Ghana, an accompanying spouse may be restricted by law from working. What do they

---

[1] *"A Call to Alms"* by David Marchese, Good Weekend, The Age, May 18, 2019.

© The Author(s), under exclusive license to Springer Nature Switzerland AG 2021
I. Howie, *Reflections on a United Nations' Career*, Springer Biographies,
https://doi.org/10.1007/978-3-030-77063-1_6

do if they have a professional career? Not all partners want to join the diplomatic circuit, play golf, frequent international clubs or take local employment at local rates. As a consequence, they may spend more and more time back in their home country, meaning a separated family, or they may remain becoming bored and dissatisfied in their large rented house complete with servants. For children, it can be equally problematic. How well I remember my daughter's first day at the Ghana International School, her fourth school in five years. She tentatively entered yet another new classroom and with tears in her eyes, looked back at me. After she disappeared into the room, I stood there for a long time feeling her pain. Months later, when I picked her up at the end of the day in the dusty school car park, I would see her chatting happily with her new friends By now she knew all the vendors selling roasted meat to the children awaiting their ride home; the "small chop" with the hot "shitto" pepper sauce. Once at home, the phone rang constantly with her conversations alternating between intimate and earnest whispers to shrieking and noisy exchanges. Her mixed racial "crowd" moved around en masse from the beach to each other's houses, to eating places and to school parties. Afro-American music and fashion dominated with the boy's "uniform" consisting of baggy shorts, baseball caps on backwards or sideways, basketball boots and a crown of black curly hair with shaved sides. But, despite the apparent integration, my daughter paid a price for the continual disruptions in those turbulent teenage years.

On arrival in Accra we stayed at the Golden Tulip Hotel, where I later joined the gym, a pattern I have followed with every posting. From the hotel, we began our search for accommodation, eventually renting a two-story house in the suburbs. Just after we moved in and were in the process of unpacking the various boxes of our shipment from Nairobi, we were burgled. While we slept, thieves climbed up to the second floor and helped themselves. This was not a good start. In retrospect, however, it was a big plus because we resolved that we would no longer stay in that house. We would look elsewhere. As a result, I came to hear of a compound that was owned by Shell. Located on a long, tree-lined avenue, it was much more central than the distant suburb where we first rented and close to the UN offices. Not only was it safer, being near to the President's home, it included a semi-circular driveway, angling through expansive grounds plus separate staff quarters. There were also two bungalows to choose from. I negotiated with Shell who agreed to our occupying one. It was a two-story house with a screened veranda to the side. It then happened that the UN Resident Coordinator (UN terminology for ambassador) agreed to rent the other bungalow as the house provided to her by the government was being repaired. The Resident

Coordinator was a single woman and we soon became very close friends.[2] This friendship was one of the joys of our time in Ghana. It typified my UN experience whereby long-term associations were made with colleagues first met on arrival.[3]

Not long after we had both moved into our respective houses, our neighbour had a visit from Flight Lieutenant Rawlings then known as the Chief Martial Law Administrator (a euphemism for a dictator). It was around 9 o'clock in the evening. She was quietly reading on the sofa prior to going to bed. Her relaxed composure was suddenly disrupted when the housekeeper rushed into tell her that the Flight Lieutenant had just driven up to the front door on his motorbike. At this time 'Jerry or JJ' was known to get around the city minus any security detail, a practice that was quickly reversed. When the UNRC received the military strongman in her sitting room, she was very puzzled, indeed nervous, as to why this surprising guest had suddenly appeared, alone and in military uniform. Over a cup of tea, he explained. The senior most court in the country had found a woman guilty of murder and condemned her to hang. The woman had then lodged a plea for clemency to the highest authority in the land, namely, the Lieutenant, and he was struggling with the decision he had to make. "Should I commute her sentence or not?" he asked our UN ambassador. "I am conflicted by the gravity of the ruling I have to make and I thought as a senior UN official, as well as a Canadian and a woman, you might be able to guide me." For the next hour or so they debated the merits and demerits of capital punishment. Then, as suddenly as he had appeared, Jerry departed out the front door, hopped on his motorbike and roared off into the night.

After the burglary and our subsequent move, the second challenge I faced related to Christmas, typically a time of joy and celebration. One day, in early December, I was informed[4] that the practice here in Accra was to welcome the festive season by buying Johnnie Walker Black Label whiskey duty-free

---

[2]Her name was Lynn Wallis, and she was a woman of great integrity, but very regrettably she was declared persona non grata when it was said she had a falling out with the First Lady. We heard about this when she contacted us in New Zealand while we were on home leave. When we returned to Accra it fell to us to pack up her household. Very sadly, she died while we were posted in China.

[3]Flight Lieutenant Rawlings became Head of State briefly in 1979. He returned to power on the 31 December 1981 and was in charge until 2001.

[4]No longer being an 'expert' on assignment meant that I did not have to recruit staff but inherited them from the previous UNFPA representative. They consisted of two secretaries, a national programme officer, a finance officer and two drivers. One of the two secretaries served as my personal assistant and proved to be a most wonderful appointment. Equally superb were the two drivers. It was with these three that I spent most of my working hours.

from the bonded warehouse,[5] and then delivering them as gifts to ministers and other senior government officials. When I enquired where the large amount of money required for this purchase came from, I was told it came from the country programme budget and not the personal account of the representative. Because the programme budget was allocated from UNFPA headquarters and was made up of the funding contributed by taxpayers throughout the world, via their government aid programmes, this was a practice I was loath to follow. I aired my reservations with the staff and was told that it would be in my best interests, as a new arrival, to extend UN generosity. Future support for our programme aspirations could well depend on it. It was a telling moment for me. I could see my undoing. I imagined a Ghanaian minister so disappointed at not receiving his dozen Black Label that at a future meeting with my UN superiors, he mentioned how dissatisfied he was with the country director for not 'properly representing' UNFPA. Corridor gossip, true or not, was and still is, a powerful aphrodisiac in many organisations. The UN was no exception. What should be my attitude now with respect to crates of whiskey? I decided I wouldn't do it. It was corrupt. I said no. The weeks leading up to Christmas were a nervous period. I expected a phone call or a whispered request at any moment asking where the the bottles were. But I didn't hear a thing. Life went on. I learnt a lesson, yet another, on how to operate and how to uphold standards of propriety applicable in any circumstance. Years later, when I became chief of human resources, I again saw the slippery slope that our representatives could be placed in and recalled my own anxiety when so positioned. Dealing with children starting a new school, then robbery and corruption were among the early baptisms by fire to my time in Accra. Now I needed to put these experiences to one side and get onto the front foot if I was going "to make a difference". But where to start and, besides, it was the holiday season. I began with a bit of reading.

As I read and observed, I came to appreciate Ghana's rich history and its highly developed culture. Although I was never consciously aware of the visual and linguistic differences between ethnic groups, I understood that the largest group were the Akan people who made up nearly half of the population. Pre-colonisation, the Akans had established a powerful nation known as *Denkyira* but they were brought to their knees by the Asante people who successfully challenged their control of the gold-mining industry. Following this, many chiefs recognised the authority of the Asante King.

---

[5]Access to duty free purchases is a common privilege accorded to diplomats the world over.

Just like Kenya, Ghana also saw Portuguese traders arriving in the late 1450s. They were searching for gold, naming the area the 'Gold Coast'. By the end of the 16th century, the area produced 10% of the world's gold. Dutch, British, and Danish settlements followed arriving in the mid-18th century. All the European conquerors engaged in the slave trade and the forts along Ghana's coastline, such as Elmina Castle and at Cape Coast, attested to the horrors of this practice.[6] When the Danes departed in 1850, the British began to take over the abandoned settlements and then they occupied the Dutch enclaves. In 1901 Britain declared the southern territory a colony by settlement, the northern territory a protectorate and Ashanti a colony by conquest. Growing national pressure for self-determination saw Britain gradually surrender its control. Known during colonial times as the 'white man's grave' because of malaria, the British were keen to extricate themselves and prepared the country for independence. The 1946 constitution required the legislative council to have an African majority, but it was after elections in 1951 that Kwame Nkrumah, a Ghanaian politician, became prime minister. Following a UN-supervised general election in May 1956, the Convention People's Party (CPP), led by Nkrumah, won with a big majority.[7] The country became independent in 1957, the first European colony in Sub-Saharan Africa to do so, and three years later became a republic with Nkrumah its first president. In 1964 it was declared a one-party state with the CPP being the sole authorised party. Less than two years later (February 1966), Ghana saw the first of four military coups. Nkrumah was removed.[8] A further three followed in 1972, 1979 and 1981. From December 1981 until November 1992 Ghana was ruled by a Provisional National Defence Council (PNDC) established by Flt-Lt Jerry J Rawlings. In 1988, he oversaw one of the most comprehensive decentralisation reforms in Africa.[9] New district assemblies were created, increasing the number from 65 to 110 by 1992. The aim was to bridge the development gap between the rural and urban areas and ensure popular participation in governance at the grassroots level. In April 1992, a draft constitution for the restoration of multiparty democracy was

---

[6]The return of the African American diaspora to Ghana has been a feature of Ghanaian life dating back decades. From W.E.B. Du Bois who settled in Ghana in the last years of his life and is buried in Accra to the estimated 3,000 African American residents most of whom live in the capital.

[7]The CPP was a socialist and nationalist political party based on the ideas of Kwame Nkrumah. It promoted a pan-African culture and played a leading role in African international relations during the decolonisation period.

[8]When Nkrumah was deposed the principal reasons cited were corruption, dictatorial practices, the deteriorating economy, and his aggressive involvement in African politics. He lived the rest of his life in Guinea.

[9]Ayee, J. R. A. 'The Political Economy of the Creation of Districts in Ghana' Journal of Asian and African Studies, Vol. 48, No. 5, pp. 623–645.

approved by referendum. The National Democratic Congress (NDC) was formed to contest the elections on behalf of the PNDC. In the November presidential election Rawlings was elected. He was sworn in as President in January 1993 when the state's military went back to barracks. This was my third year in the country. By that time and after 36 years of independence, Ghana had seen nine different types of government (three civilians and six military).

Despite its military coups Ghana seemed more politically stable, at least compared with some of its neighbours. There may have been years of economic decline but it was still spoken of as a 'lucky' country. The first to achieve independence before anyone else in the region, it had high levels of education and an economy based on industrial diamonds, cocoa, gold, mahogany, and bauxite. Since taking power, Rawlings had seen the country achieve one of the highest growth rates in Africa. Ghana, although not ethnically homogeneous, also seemed less ideologically and culturally divided than other countries, certainly when compared with Kenya. There was not the hostility towards foreigners experienced elsewhere. You were immediately accepted irrespective of your ethnicity.[10] During the three years of economic and political changes that we saw in Ghana, I watched the country assert the confidence that an identity going back centuries demanded.

Family Planning came late to sub-Saharan Africa, and in the early nineties the region continued to struggle with massive population growth, poverty,[11] limited resources and extremely high fertility. Ghana was largely cited as an exception to this scenario having the most successful family planning programme in the region. Its family planning efforts began around 1959 when President Nkrumah agreed for Ghana to take part in the 1960 round of national censuses, as proposed by the United Nations. Although as a socialist he was personally opposed to family planning programmes, the proposition to hold the first modern census in Africa was said to have appealed to his

---

[10]Evidence Jerry Rawlings himself who was the son of a Scottish father and Ghanaian mother. A former air force flight lieutenant he twice overthrew governments through coups in 1979 and 1981. He then went on to head Ghana for 20 years. He died on the 12 November 2020.

[11]The estimated incidence of poverty in Ghana was 51.7% in 1991/1992. By 2012/2013 the incidence had fallen to 24.2%, a halving of the number. This meant that Ghana achieved Millennium Development Goal 1 (MDG #1). Despite the remarkable reduction, the three regions of Northern Ghana still had very high poverty levels which actually worsened between 2012/2013 and 2016/2017. During the same period, poverty in rural Ghana also worsened while urban poverty improved. Ghana Statistical Service, 'Ghana Living Standard Survey Round 6: Poverty Profile in Ghana, 2005–2013', GSS: Accra, 2014:44 and Ghana Statistical Service 'Ghana Living Standards Survey Round 7 (GLSS7): Poverty Trends in Ghana 2005–2017', GSS: Accra 2018:17.

modernizing views.[12] In 1964, the Seven-Year Development Plan (1964–70) noted that national population growth was excessive with a total fertility rate estimated to be 7.0 births per woman. A voluntary family planning association was formed in 1967 under the name 'Planned Parenthood Associated of Ghana'. Its primary objective was to lobby for the implementation of national family planning policies and programmes. In the same year, the Ghanaian government became the first Sub-Saharan African government to sign the World Leaders Declaration on Population. By 1969 the government's first policy paper, titled Population Planning for National Progress, was produced.[13] This policy was considered so comprehensive that it was used as a model for other population policies around the world[14]. But then came the detrimental effects of the severe economic crisis experienced during the 1970s and the early 1980s. While studies in the mid-eighties revealed that the vast majority of Ghanaians knew about modern methods of contraception, just 12.8% of women were using any contraceptive and only 5.1% a modern method.[15] Economic development and quality-of-life had not increased with population growth.

In 1990 when I arrived and 21 years after enunciating a farsighted and progressive policy, the population totalled 16 million having increased more than five-fold between 1921 and 1984. Ministry of Health statistics showed that the average number of children per woman was six nationwide, but this was a drop from seven. Regional variations, however, were quite marked with the Northern Region showing an increase of 3.2% per year and the Volta Region only 1.7%. Rates were even lower in urban areas. This change was attributed, in part, to economic hardship aggravated by unsubsidised health services, high school fees and housing shortages. Ghana now stood poised to either regain the population initiative or continue its erratic record of programme performance. It needed to reinvigorate its population programme.

---

[12]Warren C. Robinson and John A. Ross, Editors, THE GLOBAL FAMILY PLANNING REVOLUTION: THREE DECADES OF POPULATION POLI CIES AND PROGRAMS. The International Bank for Reconstruction and Development/The World Bank, Washington, DC, 2007. http://siteresources.worldbank.org/INTPRH/Resources/GlobalFamilyPlanningRevolution.pdf PG379.

[13]The committee charged with drawing up the plan included two members who later I came to know well. The first was Fred T. Sai, professor of social and preventive medicine in the University of Ghana Medical School and later Senior Advisor on Population to the President of the World Bank from 1985 to 1990. The other was Dr. Gordon Perkin, one of the co-founders of the Programme for Appropriate Technology in Health (PATH) and the Gates Foundation's first director of global health.

[14]Caldwell, J. C & Sai, F. T, 2007, 'Family Planning in Ghana', in Robinson, W. C, & Ross, J. A, eds., The Global Family Planning Revolution: Three Decades of Population Policies and Programs, The World Bank: Washington D.C., pp. 379–391, available online: http://siteresources.worldbank.org/INTPRH/Resources/GlobalFamilyPlanningRevolution.pdf> [6 June 2015].

[15]1988 Demographic and Health Survey.

1990 was also a transitional one for the UNFPA programme of assistance to the government. Not only was I new but those twelve months were a conduit between the formal closure of the first country programme, 1985–1989, and the formal inauguration of the second country programme, 1991–1995 with a budget of more than US $10 million. In common with the standard UNFPA language of the time, there were several main elements to both programmes. The first came under the heading "Policy Development" and included assistance to the integration of population into development planning and strengthening the analysis and dissemination of demographic data. The second was titled "Institution Building" and sought to strengthen the national maternal and child health/family planning programme. Finally, "Community Mobilisation" aimed to support information, education and communication (IEC) activities and strengthen women's organisations in the area of population and development. What all this language meant when translated into measurable actions was not entirely clear, nor how each funded project that made up the programme was meant to work together. Also missing was any collaboration between the Fund and other international agencies working in the general area of population. So, after the initial round of appointments with key government, donor and UN colleagues, my first initiative was to bring together all the project directors in the various government departments, their UNFPA-funded international advisers along with their national counterparts, and the representatives of the various agencies working in the field of population and health. With government approval, I established a Programme Management Team (PMT).[16]

I chose the title "Programme Management Team" very carefully. I wanted all the members to think programmatically, not in terms of individual projects loosely cobbled together. I wanted them to see that we were running an interconnected programme, where working together reinforced our efforts to achieve the goals of the country programme. I called it 'management' because I wanted this team to take responsibility for their programme: managing it, monitoring performance, adjusting as required and taking ownership. It was their national programme and not one driven by foreign donors. As such, local project directors were responsible for its management. Lastly, I called it a 'team'. I chose this term to demonstrate that all the local project managers, plus their advisers and the government planning officials, were working together. Being emphasised again was back-stopping, learning

---

[16] I would have preferred the Director of the Manpower and International Cooperation Division in the Ministry of Finance and Economic Planning (essentially, my counterpart) to have initiated such meetings and held them in the government offices. I did not see my action as an appropriate role for a donor to take. When no such calls were made, I proposed that we jointly chair the meetings which were held in the UN conference room.

together, sharing resources and collective decision-making—a team working together to manage a programme including the allocation and utilisation of financial resources by each project (i.e. by annual allocation, cash expenditure ceiling by year, actual expenditure and expenditure as a % of cash ceiling). Later, we began reporting the same information to the resuscitated National Population Council and its 28 member agencies. This council was the government's highest advisory body and assumed responsibility for all policy and planning related to population activities.[17]

One of the first exercises of the "team" was to examine what we actually knew about Ghanaians' reproductive and contraceptive knowledge and practice. Until we actually knew what was going on, how could we decide what we needed to do? We wanted a starting-point and later we found we had to have this reference to monitor progress and evaluate. The starting point chosen was the 1984 census. In collaboration with the Canadian International Development Agency (CIDA), UNFPA financed the purchase of computers and printers and then the training of government statisticians and computer programmers. The government could now analyse the data and disseminate the results. With this information plus that of other surveys we published a 14-page booklet titled "UNFPA in Ghana. Together since 1972—Partners into the Future". In this we outlined Ghana's demographic profile, notably its population size, growth and age structure and the accompanying socio-economic implications. We included a summary of the government's population policy as well as a chart of the national family-planning programme, including a list of local and international partners who were working in the country. We referred to the limited achievements so far realised, and the constraints that gave rise to these, but wanting to be positive, we explained how, since 1985 and the reinvigoration of the national family-planning programme, Ghana had been fortunate to have a multi-sectoral programme supported by many agencies. It was also fortunate, we wrote, in having political leadership committed to reducing future rates of population growth. Indeed, it was the CMLA and now President, Jerry Rawlings, who asked me directly, "Why has it taken so long to register even an

---

[17]A comparable initiative to our PMT within the broader donor community working in the health and population sector at this time, was the launching of a monthly donor meeting. The meeting was chaired by the World Bank and co-chaired by UNDP. As well as reporting on what they were doing, agencies agreed a more focused approach would occur if each of us coordinated and collaborated. One example of this was an undertaking to divide the country geographically into areas of interest in order to complement each other's work and avoid overlap. For example, where the World Bank was providing the financial resources to establish a hospital, including bricks and mortar and the equipment, WHO would aim to provide the technical training to the local health officials. Another initiative was an evaluation of the transport system of the MOH. Over time we discovered that while complementing each other was good donors needed to avoid 'balkanisation' by choosing favoured parts of the country.

extremely moderate decrease in our rate of population growth and what did we now need to do about it?" He did so in Bolgatanga, close to the border of Burkina Faso when he presided over a rally in support of family planning.[18] Unique among African leaders at that time, Rawlings gave the family planning movement of Ghana his political commitment, as did his wife, Nana Rawlings.[19]

Despite this political support our team agreed that we needed to begin with the underlying socio-economic and cultural patterns if we wanted to have an impact on the demographic agendas. In 1987, the Brundtland Report[20] had stated that studying population without context made no sense because there were so many factors involved. Towards our understanding of the Ghanaian context, I engaged a leading researcher from the Population Council to work in collaboration with social researchers from the University of Ghana. Their UNFPA-funded Ghana Universities Press publication titled, "Family and Development in Ghana", confirmed that one of the key factors that was very hard to determine let alone measure, was cultural and collective change. There were clearly socio-cultural factors that were barriers to contraception. Birth spacing was widely viewed as birth stopping. Many men still equated large families with prestige, wealth, and security, and they feared that contraception would enable their partners to become "promiscuous flirts". Not only was husband/wife communication minimal but contraceptive use was often mistaken for abortion and thus condemned.

---

[18]In a letter to my parents I described this launch of family planning week. "Right now," I wrote, "I am on the official dais awaiting the arrival of the president. A heavily armed commando stands guard next to me. Out on the parade ground, groups of drummers are dancing. The public address system is blaring out instructions. It announces the chiefs who enter the square in flowing robes protected from the glaring sun by nobles holding large umbrellas. As they enter, the drummers start up again swirling back-and-forth on the ground before us. Women give loud yodelling calls. The men twist to face each other hitting sticks together in rhythm. Quite a sight. And, all for family planning!"

[19]First Lady Nana Konadu Agyeman Rawlings was one of our key project partners. She had become president of the 31st December Women's Movement in 1982. Since then, the movement has established day-care centres and nurseries, bakeries, fishing cooperatives for women, food-processing factories and a host of economic programmes. It raised money from both the government and the United Nations' agencies including UNFPA. I came to appreciate the movement's ability to organise women and channel programmes of social change, including literacy and family planning, through their rural network. The Rawlings were not without their critics nor their enemies, especially over the way power had been seized, but to their credit they had been outspoken in their support of family planning. This was unique among African leaders and I, for one, welcomed it. Nana Rawlings was fun to travel with as were her team and the village rallies, I attended were a riot of colour, singing and dancing. Politics and party largesse may have been the motivation, but they were, typically, grass root dialogues about matters that mattered to rural women.

[20]The Brundtland Report was published after the successful World Commission on Environment and Development in 1987. It was named after former Norwegian PM, Gro Harlem Brundtland, and notably addressed the urgent need for environmental sustainability in development initiatives. United Nations, Commission on Sustainable Development, "Framing Sustainable Development: The Brundtland Report", April 1987.

Reinforcing this challenging environment were marked regional variations (something the UN rarely talks of, preferring global inequalities). We knew that the north of the country was still under served when compared with the south. In 1988 the Ministry of Health had created a research centre in Navrongo, the capital of Kassena-Nankana District in the Upper East Region, with the mandate to investigate health problems of the Sahelian ecological belt of northern Ghana and advise policymakers. The study district was rural, dispersedly populated and remote. Published findings revealed that in this part of the country, traditions and practices restricted women's autonomy and the introduction of family planning. Compounding the situation was a very low female literacy rate which increased women's dependence on men and reinforced gender stratification. Prevailing customs such as bride wealth and polygamy endorsed the perception of women as property purchased by the extended family to produce children. The social, economic, and geographic circumstances of northern Ghana also constrained health service delivery and, thus, the provision of family planning services. The lack of resources for outreach programmes (vehicles, fuel, and staff) limited the provision of outreach care, and the cost of travel to clinics was prohibitive for many families.

This northern situation was made very clear to me on an early visit to a major regional hospital. I saw patients lying on the floor, with the infectious and non-infectious lumped together. There was virtually no equipment, and few drugs. The bed fittings were rusted with three babies sharing a crib. It was the responsibility of families to bring their sick relatives' food most of which was purchased in the nearby market along with the drugs and blood which were also on sale. Regrettably, most of the young interns told me that they would, on graduation, leave the country. They were not paid enough, they said, and when it did come, it came irregularly.[21] Despite this and the crowds cramming every ward, we were always welcomed with the doctors following the procedures they had inherited from their British training.

---

[21] In 1990 there were no more doctors in the country than there were in 1970. 23 years of medical graduates had virtually all emigrated. In 2017 it was estimated there were 700 Ghanaian doctors in the United States. Such an exodus meant that within Ghana the ratio of doctors to population was 1 per 15,000 in 2010 (compared with 1 per 300 in Australia). Exacerbating the situation was the exodus of skilled midwives. As fast as the country produced them, able to manage complicated pregnancies and avert maternal deaths, they were on the first plane out to change bedpans in geriatric homes for a 20 fold increase in salary above what they could earn from the Ministry of Health. In the early nineties we suggested a two-pronged approach—quadruple output from midwifery schools and offer substantial benefits above salaries so that the midwives would remain in Ghana. Today, to rectify this situation the Government has increased the salaries of doctors, offered post graduate training, regionalised medical colleges, and decentralised postings. As a result of these efforts, by 2014 the ratio had fallen to 1 in 8,500.

In 1990, then, the challenges faced were formidable. Our two widely disseminated booklets were useful in giving UNFPA a starting profile but our PMT knew that, in the final analysis, family planning issues needed to be discussed and decided upon between couples, between men and women many of whom were rural based and semi-literate. To achieve such behavioural change within the five-year time frame of a UNFPA programme was impossible, especially when it came to empowering women. Still, our team agreed to a strategy that if we were to achieve the goals we set, we must not repeat the disappointments of the past. The goals included addressing supply-side constraints, increased emphasis on the quality and continuity of client care, addressing underserved populations such as men and adolescents, decentralising management capacity to sub-district level along integrated lines rather than by vertical divisions, increasing awareness of and support for longer-lasting contraceptive methods and deepening political commitment to the national policy. Having taken the pulse via our situational analyses, it was in the increased supply of contraceptives where I saw our greatest impact. UNFPA had, very fortuitously, engaged the technical services of the Royal Tropical Institute (KIT in Dutch) to work with the far-sighted leadership of the MCH Division in the Ministry of Health. It began with their acceptance that sexual and reproductive health care was a major component of primary health care services in a district. Women, men and adolescents needed quality information and services to allow them to have a safe and fulfilling sexual and reproductive life. For this to happen, the project launched a six-step framework of activities and processes to support action at the national, provincial and district level: 1. collaborative planning, programming and resource allocation; 2. strategic assessment; 3. policy and strategy development; 4. development of guidelines/materials; 5. RH programme management; and 6. policy review. Because there was political leadership and, most importantly, inspired direction within the MCH division, the Ministry of Health owned the project and were prepared to scale up their initial efforts if they were successful. It was also known that information and services on sexual and reproductive health and rights needed to be gender-sensitive and culturally appropriate and that, to the extent possible, women and their communities needed to be active and equitable participants in deciding RH priorities. So it was that on the basis of these underlying premises, UNFPA in 1991 supported the implementation of a supply-side strategy with 3 modern methods of family planning and trained suppliers in 110 districts. For this, midwifery and safe motherhood skills had to be upgraded in every health facility of the country. Our partners were the Ministry of Health, USAID who supplied about 85% of the ministry's contraceptives, the Ghana Social

Marketing Programme (a USAID initiative), the local IPPF affiliate, Planned Parenthood Association of Ghana, the Ghana Registered Midwives Association and the Traditional Birth Attendant Support Project. The projected numbers to be involved ran into thousands.

A framework for in-service training for every midwife was then prepared by Johns Hopkins University and institutionalised nationwide.[22] This included the preparation of national clinical and operational protocols via a pioneering record keeping and accountability system that was later upgraded to a workable MIS. Also included as part of community-based distribution were traditional birth attendants (TBAs), district FP field assistants attached to the Department of Social Welfare and traditional healers. When we were told that lack of transport was limiting the outreach effectiveness of these various field staff, UNFPA funded the purchase of motor bikes with Save the Children Fund (SCF) providing the maintenance and spare parts and the WB and UNDP additional logistic support. A 10-year timeframe was allocated to this package of endeavours and important to its sustainability was our financing of fellowships for regional medical officers to the Liverpool School of Tropical Medicine. And, most significantly, they all returned at the end of their master's degrees.

By 1993, the results of these initiatives were impressive. The number of service delivery points expanded, while contraceptive use rose so dramatically (couple years of protection increased by almost 700% with a total contraceptive prevalence near to 18%) that we had a contraceptive shortfall for which I approved a supplementary budget to purchase more supplies. DFID also came to our aid with an allocation of UK£1 million with which to buy contraceptives. In summary, the sharpest recorded decline in total fertility in African history was achieved in Ghana from 1989 to 1994 for which UNFPA was at the cutting edge.

---

[22]Supported by the American College of Midwives and Family Care International Ann Starrs.

Chronology of HMIS interventions in Ghana and family planning performance indicators (1976–93).[23]

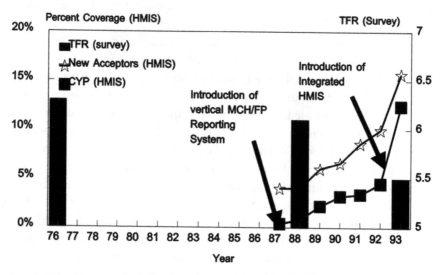

Source: National Survey Data: WFS 1976, DHS 1988 and 1993; and HMIS 1987-1993

Ghana 1993: Results from the Demographic and Health Survey Studies in Family Planning. Vol 26. No 4. July/August. 1995. The Population Council. New York. NY. USA and HMIS data.

Of course, there were many hiccups along the way. Early on we saw that the substantial effort our team was making to collect data from a multiplicity of sources was not serving its intended function. It was realised that even when the raw data was perfect there was no point collating it simply as an end in itself. All too often it was a "box ticking" exercise but numbers never speak for themselves. Without utilisation and analysis, they were irrelevant. Like the production of audio-visual materials, they had to serve a purpose beyond the actual production. Initially, our Ghanaian efforts were too small. They provided little to no information about programme performance, let alone the impact on people's lives, and they failed to explain why and how programmes performed as they did—evidence which could be used to improve operational decisions. We also often ended up with more data than we could manage. Over time, however, because of the regional and district reporting mechanisms that were introduced, the data submitted by our Ministry of Health midwives at their quarterly planning meetings became substantial. The MCH Division eventually had all the required metrics to

---

[23]Ghana 1993: Results from the Demographic and Health Survey Studies" in Family Planning. Vol 26. No 4. July/August. 1995. The Population Council. New York. NY. USA and HMIS data.

make costings (evidence the calculation that the cost of delivering one Couple Year of Protection (CYP) was US$ 11–12[24]). But this was not enough. Even though it took time and effort to produce these calculations they served no use if the trends shown were confined only to the producers. We resolved to place the results before our implementing partners, our UNFPA programme management team, other donors and ultimately the government. And, here, we made a most significant intervention. We presented the data to the government at budget time. Result? The government committed its <u>own</u> funds to overcome a contraceptive supply shortfall.

Concurrent to this unique drive from the Ministry of Health there were the more standard interventions that made up the UNFPA/Government programme. As I travelled around the country listening to people, I found that their perceptions of family planning were influenced by rumour and superstition. In Greater Accra, the Dangme people told me that family planning was dangerous and that the best contraceptive was saccharin. In common with many others they said that using contraception was part of flirting and promiscuity, and that condoms meant men losing control. In Berekum town in the centre of the country, there was a widespread belief the government wanted to stop people having children. "*Twa awo*" was the often-used expression literally meaning 'having your womb turned'. In other words, sterilisation, stop having children, enough. Further north in Bolga, the regional capital of Upper East, a common refrain was that if "government ('those officials in Mitsubishi Pajeros') wanted us to practise family planning, then let it guarantee our children won't die". There was so much hearsay and rumours in this region that family planning had a very bad name. It was common to think it caused infertility, sickness, abortion, early menopause, dizziness, bleeding and castration. People were not only shy but afraid when the subject was mentioned. The government needed a national IEC policy to address the rumours and hearsay and to simply explain what family planning was and how it could benefit individuals, especially those teenage mothers, couples and when used lead to healthy children.

The national 1993 Health Behaviour Change Strategy sought to address many of these misconceptions via defining target audiences, setting a desired behaviour, stating what the current level of FP practice was, declaring a desired level of practice and how that level needed to be measured. Towards implementing this strategy, we supported Christian and Muslim family counselling services, and used folk media to communicate family planning

---

[24]During all my years with UNFPA this was the only occasion I saw this key indicator of the success of a family planning programme utilised. As a point of comparison, Marie Stopes International, a global provider of SRH services, calculated in 2019 that it cost UK£7 per CYP. MSI makes this calculation both as proof of its effectiveness and as a key budget control measure.

messages, approaches which I had used so successfully in Bangladesh. Given the youth bulge in the population we also supported peer counselling in reproductive health for adolescents. AIDS was now an emerging crisis and following my participation in an analysis of the population challenges faced by Botswana I saw how this scourge could devastate a country and how a well-governed country sought to deal with it. A national strategy for Ghana was soon developed. Assisting us, as they did in many things, were a team of Ghanaian demographers most of whom had studied at the Australian National University under the guidance of the distinguished demographer Professor Jack Caldwell.

While UNFPA was operating on a national scale, as a collaborative partner of the government, I was witness during these years in Ghana to a grassroots initiative that demonstrated what local commitment, devoid of fanfare, could achieve. It began with our neighbour, a Canadian family. Each afternoon when the four children returned from school the mother would sit with them on their veranda and read stories. Before long the children of her neighbours, including our young son, would join and they would all sit listening. Initially there were six children and a basket of books. Very quickly, the reading circle expanded until there were 75 children in the garden. Clearly, there was a desire among Ghanaian children to read books. To make space for more children, the family turned its guest room into a tiny library and trained their housekeeper to be the first librarian. They called this fledgling library the Osu Community Library because it was located on Osu Avenue. To support its functioning, they also founded a non-profit Ghanaian charity named the Osu Library Fund. More books were purchased along with small tables and chairs and a university student was engaged to read to the children and to listen as they read their books. Because of the growing numbers, a 40-foot shipping container was purchased for US$1,200. Windows and a door were cut out, floors and ceiling fans painted bright blue and colourful cushions and wall hangings added. In the words of Kathy, the founder, "We wanted our library to be beautiful so we planted a garden with bright pink bougainvillea bushes outside the doors". The new library was opened on November 13, 1992. Second-hand books were then scoured from all over the world and a local librarian engaged. Within three months you could see the children line up, select their book and then place it in a cloth bag which the library provided and which helped them not only carry their book but also care for it. Today, these two Osu organisations have built eight large community libraries mainly in impoverished parts of the Greater Accra region and have helped to create more than 200 libraries in Africa, mainly small-scale initiatives in schools and rural communities. Thousands of children have joined as members and if you walk into any of these libraries on any afternoon, you will find them packed with eager children, all of them reading or interacting in the puzzle room. Additionally, as the children have turned into teenagers there are now performance spaces for theatre groups and for other cultural activities. One of the libraries in Accra has a scholarship fund which provides school fees and uniforms for deserving library members. It also has a bathing programme, and a food programme where a hot meal is served to 30 children daily. They even have a women's soccer team, and since 1994 have offered free literacy classes twice weekly for those who have never attended school. And it all began on our neighbour's veranda. I highlight the Osu library not just because it is a success story but because it is an example of one determined woman's response to a need who then scaled it up through local institution building, a goal to be found in every UN programme document.[25] Commitment, continuity, local financing, local staff and the ability to navigate government pressures explain this extraordinary achievement.

Throughout our nearly four years in Accra, the highlight of our week was the Sunday we spent as a family on the beach at what was locally known as "Mile 16".[26] Along with others we rented space from the local chief for an annual price of a bottle of Arak. We built a thatched hut at the edge of the sand and furnished it with a wooden table and bench. Countless visitors were invited to have lunch, to walk on the beach and occasionally to risk swimming in the very choppy water. On our return to town we often stopped at a school for music where the so named master was teaching African drumming to a group of young men. Their playing was exquisite. Using long narrow drumsticks or their hands they would rhythmically and rapidly tap softly or loudly and hold us entranced for an hour at the end of a hot and sultry day. I have heard multiple performances of African drumming since but never heard the equal of those performances. An associated highlight revolved around the return of the African American diaspora to their slave roots in Ghana. These were often well-known entertainment figures and included Dionne Warwick, Isaac Hayes and Public Enemy, the well-known rap group who gave a concert at the Portuguese castle in Cape Coast built to house the slaves captured in the hinterland before their shipment to the Americas.

---

[25]There are multiple examples of successful small-scale projects throughout the developing world. Often pioneered by very committed people with support from individuals and church groups in their home countries they contribute mightily to the improved well-being of the poor. Where Osu is different is that it went beyond a strictly local initiative to a national and even international institution.

[26]The only weekends when we limited our trips to "Mile 16" were during the extremes of the annual Harmattan season. From the end of November to the middle of March a dry and dusty north easterly trade wind blew from the Sahara Desert over the West African subcontinent. The sky would darken with clouds of dust. The sun would disappear, down would come the temperature and gone, for the moment, was the humidity. At times during the height of the season you couldn't even see the front gate.

It was while attending a regional meeting of UNFPA country directors in Dhaka, Senegal, in March 1993, that the possibility of reassignment to China was raised. It was common practice at such meetings for representatives to seek an appointment with the Executive Director. During my appointment, she surprised me by asking where I would like to be assigned next. I then surprised myself by declaring China. I had never been to the country nor knew anything much of its family planning programme. What further motivation did I need? Did I know anything of the global politics surrounding the programme? Not really. It was just a "put it out there" nomination. In the absence of any vacancy announcement, there the matter rested.

Later that month I received a call from the Director of the Africa Division of the Fund, the only one I ever received from him, asking if I would like to be reassigned to China with non-residential responsibilities for North Korea and Mongolia. "Yes" I said, "But not yet. I have a substantial programme here in Ghana for which I am responsible, and I want to complete it." He agreed to a delay, and I had my first lesson in the power of negotiation. I discovered you weren't as beholden to arbitrary decisions coming from Headquarters as I thought. You could actually pick and choose assignments, lobby for them, and nominate the timing that suited you best. Welcome to the system. For a slow learner, I was becoming aware of "The Knowledge" (i.e., knowing the dividing line between a caring organisation and how to work the system to your advantage).

Timing for the transfer later in the year was eventually agreed to, the family alerted and the usual relocation initiatives begun. And, there, for the moment, the matter rested. Well, not quite. I learned later that President Rawlings, was not pleased that I was being transferred out of his country. During a visit by the New York based-UNDP Administrator Rawlings had asked him why they were withdrawing me. Later, in early July 1993, I was called to the President's office in the Osu Castle, the official seat of government, to receive his personal thanks. Then, immediately following the national launching of family population and planning week in Bolgatanga, which I attended in the presence of the President , his Special Assistant wrote to UNFPA's Executive Director as follows:

The President would like me to express his appreciation of the immense contribution that the United Nations Population Fund is making to the achievement of our population control objectives.

He has been particularly impressed with the dynamism and commitment of your Country Director, Mr Ian Howie who is doing a remarkable work in Ghana.

The President has however learned with regret that Mr Howie is being posted to another assignment. He would very much appreciate if Mr Howie's tour could be extended to enable him to help in stepping up the momentum of our population activities now taking off.[27]

I knew nothing of the letter at the time, and it was many years later that I first saw it when accessing my personal file at UNFPA Headquarters. No reply was shown and there may not have been one. As I was to discover, such letters from a national leader were often viewed with suspicion at headquarters, the thinking being that the concerned staff member may have manipulated its writing in the hope of achieving some advantage or avoiding a reassignment. When in Ghana I never knew such was possible. If I had known, I would never have attempted to do so.

There was a second challenge the Executive Director faced concerning my appointment (at least from my perspective). It came from the Administrator of UNDP who asked her if I could be released to join UNDP as a Resident Representative (a UNDP Res Rep as was commonly referred to). "Oh no, I wouldn't agree to that" the ED told me later when recounting the story, "we need him to continue with us!" Had I known at the time, I may well have considered the opportunity and my UN career would have taken a different path.

A third surprising turn of events also awaited my China posting, which again, I only discovered by accident. In late May, I received a call from a friend working for an international NGO. She enquired whether I had seen the article on the front page of the New York Times informing the reader that UNFPA was thinking of withdrawing from China. "No, I hadn't", I replied, astonished. Living in Accra, I was not a daily reader of the Times or even an intermittent one. Nor had anyone from headquarters ever hinted that UNFPA was thinking of exiting China. As far as I knew, I was on target for reassignment later in the year. Being in the dark, I went to the source of the story.

On May 15, 1993, Nicholas Kristof, then the New York Times correspondent in Beijing, wrote:

Alarmed by indications of a harsh family planning crackdown in the Chinese countryside, the United Nations Population Fund is considering withdrawing from China and ending its work in the most populous country in the world.

The Fund's withdrawal…would end a fierce decade-long controversy about the role of the United Nations in China's one-child family planning program. The Population Fund has become associated—unfairly, many diplomats say— with the forced sterilizations and other coercive measures that China uses to

---

[27]Letter to the ED from the Special Assistant to the President, 13 July 1993.

control its population growth...peasants say the authorities routinely swoop down on villages and forcibly sterilize women who have filled their 'quota' of one or two births."[28]

That no-one at UNFPA saw fit to inform me that a withdrawal from China was a distinct possibility indicated a lack of professionalism from both the programme's side and from a human resources' perspective. Of course, the Executive Director denied the Kristof story, saying withdrawal was never mentioned, but rumour had it the reporter stood by his account having recorded the conversation. And there, for me at least, the story died. No one from the Fund ever spoke to me about the news item. We were still on our way to China. We had a wonderful farewell party at our house. Many people came. Foreigners, locals, and everyone danced the night away. Ghana may have been divided economically but it was not racially or ethnically. We were always welcomed in their country as guests.

As with all my earlier assignments, I learnt a great deal by 'doing' in Ghana. Now, as a first-time representative I was also learning from others, be it the skilled development technicians at USAID or the World Bank or our own project experts from KIT. Looking back, what was significant during those years was that we had a multisectoral programme supported by many agencies within each sector, and in having political leadership committed to reducing future rates of population growth. By 1999, results indicated that significant fertility decline arose in the early years of our programme, associated as it was with the combination of services provided by community nurses and social mobilization.

But what is the situation today? By regional standards, Ghana has done modestly well. Despite cuts in foreign aid in the aftermath of the cold war (many African countries were paying more in interest than they received in aid), Ghana had been a top performer on hunger, cutting the rate by 75% since 1990 and halving the rate of child malnutrition.[29] In 2018 it was located in the lower ranks of middle income countries with a per capita income of US$4,600.[30] What of reproductive health? The TFR for the country has fallen substantially from 6 when I arrived in 1990 to 4.5 in

---

[28] Kristof D. Nicholas, 'A U.N. Agency May Leave China Over Coercive Population Control', New York Times, May 15, 1993, Accessed September 13, 2015, http://www.nytimes.com/1993/05/15/world/a-un-agency-may-leave-china-over-coercive-population-control.html.

[29] Madeleine Bunting "Equality is the one item nobody wants on the UN agenda next week" The Guardian 14 September 2010.

[30] This compares with US$39,000 in South Korea according to the International Monetary Fund. Ghana after Aid, David Pilling "The grand vision to stand alone", Financial Times Special Report, October 8, 2018.

2016, which was an achievement, but contraceptive prevalence rates (% of women aged 15–49 using a contraceptive) in the same year remained low at 30.6%.[31] A disappointing result given that this was the same figure we aimed to achieve by 1996 based on the CYP results we had recorded from 1990 to 1992. Why the poor result? Perhaps it was because our UNFPA/KIT colleagues, along with the Director of the MCH Department, all moved on (reassignments to other countries and recruitment to the UN being the explanations). The loss of this leadership with new personnel taking over meant a reduction in any scaled-up operations aimed at long-term impact. As party political priorities changed, there was also a lack of social mobilization. Perhaps this reflected a donor- driven priority that became muted once budget support shifted from a sector wide approach (e.g. one focused on health) to general budget support which would be allocated according to party manifestos. Government commitment to reducing population growth rates has waned as well. Population policy is no longer highlighted. The current President, Nana Akufo Addo, does not give it the priority it received during Rawling's time. Thus, the muted response to the alarming annual increase of 700,000–800,000.[32]

Regrettably, also, regional disparities continued to be exacerbated by population challenges. Survey data from the three northern Sahel regions suggested that unmet need for contraception continued to exist, but that demand for fertility regulation was focused on a desire to space rather than limit childbearing, meaning there had not been a sustained demographic transition. For example, the Upper West region with Wa as its capital about which in the nineties we were so concerned, is still not only the poorest in the country, it also has the largest household sizes.[33] Modern contraceptive prevalence rates remained low in these regions due to continuing sociocultural perceptions and an uneven capacity to deliver services.[34] The current UNFPA Country

---

[31] According to the World Bank collection of development indicators, compiled from officially recognized sources.

[32] Jamila Akweley Okertchiri "How Ghana's Rapid Population Growth Could Become an Emergency and Outpace Both Food Production and Economic Growth." Into Press Service, Accra and Donkorkrom, August 17, 2018.

[33] Ghana Living Standards Survey (GLSS) Round 6 Report. The report states in Page 4 that: *"Average household sizes that are higher than the national average are found in the three northern regions (5.5 for Upper West, 5.4 for Northern and 4.5 for Upper East)"* Ghana Statistical Service, Accra, 2014, page: 4.

[34] Northern Region (10.8 per cent) and Ashanti Region (20.8 per cent).

Programme, (2018–2022),[35] which is the seventh, highlighted the disparities by age, education and wealth across regions by pointing out that skilled delivery rates ranged from 92.1 per cent in the Greater Accra Region to 36.4 per cent in the northern region.[36] As a result, Ghana did not achieve its Millennium Development Goal 5 target of reducing maternal mortality to 190 per 100,000 live births.

In light of this perceived official indifference, the National Population Council called on the government in 2018 to legislate that only three children would be eligible for government financial support, and that any more children born thereafter would not qualify. It was necessary, the Council said, to bring the TFR down to 2.2.[37] This was not surprising when you consider that the current population is 29.6 million; double what it was in 1990 when I arrived. Despite the president declaring that it was not right that a "….country like Ghana, 60 years after independence, to still have its health and education budget being financed on the basis of generosity and charity of (donors)…",[38] there are still 26 UN agencies working in the health and education sectors along with multiple other partners (40 acknowledged in the Ghana Family Planning Costed Implementation Plan 2016–2020, September 2015). Amidst its very detailed assessment and costed plans I didn't see any mention in this USAID-funded 177-page report of overlap, duplication or repetition. As I read it, I wondered if any of the authors had ever heard of the very detailed UNFPA-financed regional transport policy prepared by the Ministry of Health in 1993 or the pioneering work "From data to decision making in health The evolution of a health management information system" by Sam Adjei and Charlotte Gardner, both distinguished Gahanaians, and Bruce Campbell and Arthur Heywood, UNFPA advisors or "Family And Development In Ghana" edited by Elizabeth Ardayfio-Schandorf in 1994, a joint Ghana University/UNFPA publication. These publications were 20 years old when this 2015 implementation plan was published, and it may be unreasonable to expect them to have been acknowledged. But to those

---

[35] United Nations Population Fund Country programme document for Ghana: Proposed indicative UNFPA assistance: $20.4 million: $7.8 million from regular resources and $12.6 million through co-financing modalities and/or other resources, including regular resources. Programme period: Five years. The programme will build a health system capacity to deliver voluntary family planning, midwifery and basic EmONC services to respond to the Ghana Family Planning 2020 commitments; reduce regional disparities in skilled attendance at birth; and increase the number and distribution of primary facilities providing basic EmONC. First regular session, 22–26 January 2018, New York, Item 6 of the provisional agenda UNFPA—Country programmes and related matters.

[36] In a January 1993 letter to my parents I cited a UNFPA financed study in the north of the country which recorded 860 maternal deaths per 100,000 live births. I then made the comparison with 8 in the USA.

[37] BBC World Service, 2 August 2018.

[38] Pilling op cit.

of us who worked in Ghana during the early nineties these were important pioneering works. They made a difference. The data bore that out. We measured a positive change in couple of years of protection, adolescent birth rates and met-need for family planning. Is that the case now? On paper, the current UNFPA programme is essentially what it was during my time. The same categorisations, the same financial divisions, although larger, and the same partners. Unlike the Osu Library which has gone from strength to strength without any fanfare, the UNFPA country office today highlights the delivery of its assistance to the rural poor via photos of an urban-educated élite (which, given the diminished family planning record of the government in recent years, is a practice that is clearly not working). What does this tell us about UN assistance and more broadly, the development industry? I didn't struggle with such questions immediately following Ghana and really didn't confront them again until I was posted to Viet Nam, some twelve years later. It was 1993 then and we were moving to China.

7

The Population Challenge: China

"The best time to plant a tree was twenty years ago. The second-best time is now". Chinese proverb

We arrived in Beijing in August 1993. As a family, we were better prepared for this transition. We were pleased with our geographic proximity to Australia, the international schools' programmes on offer, and the prospect of working on a challenging programme. So, instead of being innocently self-reliant and coping as best we could, we asked for some briefing in advance. To our surprise, headquarters were amenable to a pre-assignment visit en route to our final home leave from Ghana.[1] For this, my first visit to Beijing, we stayed at a hotel close to the canal which ran past the UN compound that included the offices of the UN Resident Coordinator, UNDP, UNFPA and UNIDO. Their location at the beginning of the large diplomatic enclave reflected the regard in which the UN was held. To one side of the compound and across the divided highway teeming with cars, buses and bikes was the Lufthansa Centre, the flower market and the hustle and bustle of everyday life. To the other side, settled amongst the greenery, were the embassies, the

---

[1] Compared with others, we saw ourselves as slow learners when it came to be utilising and, in some cases but not ours, manipulating the UN reassignment system to one's advantage. As I discovered, foreign embassies didn't operate like this. They spend time preparing their staff for an assignment. Months of preliminary briefings, language studies, arranged furnished accommodation on arrival, employment for accompanying spouses, prearranged linkages with the predecessor and their family, an amount of local currency for use immediately on arrival, airport reception and then transport to your pre-booked hotel. Previously, no one had ever told us to ask for such support and, so, not expecting it, we were never disappointed when none was offered.

© The Author(s), under exclusive license to Springer Nature
Switzerland AG 2021
I. Howie, *Reflections on a United Nations' Career*, Springer Biographies,
https://doi.org/10.1007/978-3-030-77063-1_7

ambassadorial residences and the high walls separating one compound from another. At the entrance to each stood a military guard 24/7 not just for our protection but also to ensure no unsolicited Chinese intrusion.

Prior to this posting I was relatively uninformed about China's policies on reproductive health. This lead me to develop the habit of taking a notebook to meetings and recording proceedings. The Chinese were very literal in their recollection of what was said, and so my lack of Mandarin language skills meant I had to be ready to recall the English translation accurately. Data, too, was key. The family planning statistics proudly declared by provincial and county level officials needed to be recorded to understand what was really going on. Over time, note-taking became second nature to me. Most of the information contained in these pages comes from these detailed notes with the intention of shedding some light on the little-known corners of the family planning picture. Despite all that has been written and said about the China family planning programme, including what some believe is the questionable role UNFPA has played in its promotion, much is still unknown.

When I took up the post our family moved into a three-bedroom apartment vacated by my predecessor and his wife. On first viewing, we were taken aback. We were on the seventh floor in one of the twelve dirty and dreary grey buildings that made up *Jianguomenwai*, one of the four diplomatic compounds in Beijing where the authorities required us to live.[2] Compared with our expansive tree-filled acreage in Accra, this was a shock. Would the children play in that squalid children's nursery area? Would we enjoy a Friday night drink in that rather rundown bar? What about the pollution, the endless grey skies, the cars parked everywhere[3] and the incessant din of the traffic that ran along the Ring Road bordering the west side of the block? But everything is relative. Soon we came to realise that our predecessors had done us a big favour by locating our new home in the quietest and sunniest

---

[2]There were four diplomatic compounds open to foreigners in Beijing at the time: Qi Jia Yuan, Jianguomenwai, Sanlitun and Tayuan. Unlike today, there was no commercial real estate which foreigners could rent. *Jianguomenwai* was controlled by the Diplomatic Services Bureau (commonly known as the s DSB to the residents) and located at the junction of Chang'an Avenue and the Second Ring Road in Beijing's Chaoyang District. It was constructed in 1971 as China's first international office and residence compound for the overseas staff of embassies, international organisations, and news agencies. During our time its four walls were guarded by armed DSB paramilitaries and we often wondered whether they were posted to monitor us going out (especially, those international news correspondents who shared the complex) or to prevent outsiders from coming in (which they didn't do all that well as evidenced by the number of foreign journalists who managed to slip through the net).

[3]Including the Ferrari owned by a very wealthy Chinese who had "managed", by one means or another, to find accommodation within the diplomatic enclave.

part of the compound. Moreover, we could move in immediately and did not have to queue for accommodation. With basic cooking and furniture necessities borrowed from the New Zealand embassy, we camped out while awaiting the arrival of our container from Accra.

We made many close friends in that large but confined foreign community. The children could meet their new friends and roam freely about the compound. The "TGIF" (Thank God it's Friday) evening gathering at the so-called Italian restaurant within our compound, became a highlight. Many friends and family came to stay. Our close proximity to Tiananmen Square meant they could borrow our bikes to explore the city. Nearby was Ritan Park complete with the opera singers, bird cages, tai chi and ballroom dancing enthusiasts, and the odd sword fighter. The 'hard' currency Friendship Store was close by as was the International Club 9 where I could get a hair cut. Mr. Wang, located in his tiny shop outside the main gate of the compound, seemed always able to cater to our basic western style food requirements. We gathered regularly with our friends at the "Jumping Fish" a very local restaurant in the midst of a busy market, so named by the children who one day had spotted a fish jump out of the tank. Other regular weekend outings and picnics we enjoyed were to the unexcavated Ming Tombs and the less populated stretches of the Great Wall. For our fitness and to supplement our local bike rides, there were regular visits to the gym at the Swissotel.

Unlike earlier project assignments where I had to recruit my own staff but comparable to Accra, a full team awaited me in the Beijing office. Our office included two other international staff—a deputy representative who was crucial for our Mongolian and North Korean programmes, and the only internationally appointed secretary to a representative throughout the entire UNFPA country office system. He was officially there because of a perceived need for confidentiality. But many thought it had more to do with the nationality he shared with the Executive Director. Perhaps questionable were his fundamentalist religious beliefs which often contradicted the values on which UNFPA was founded. Even so, he was a fine shorthand typist and a very kind man. In the course of my five year appointment, four other international staff members were contracted.[4] A further three international project advisers, already resident and funded by the programme, provided support to the Ministry of Health on gender matters and to an

---

[4]Among the contracted staff were two Junior Professional Officers (JPOs), one from Norway and the other from The Netherlands plus a Pakistani student of Chinese at a Beijing university. The student had initially volunteered in our office but then became a paid staff member so impressive was her performance. Later, another short term consultant joined us on secondment from UNHQ New York.

FAO-executed project supporting income generation activities for women. An additional staff member was later appointed following an intervention by the Australian Government requesting that one of their nationals be located within our office to monitor Australian aid to the programme, although this was not believed to be the real reason. At that time, the balance of power in the Australian Senate was held by an independent member, Brian Harradine, who was avowedly 'pro-life' (i.e. anti-abortion), a staunch Catholic and part of a global network opposed to UNFPA. Senator Harradine insisted that if Australia were to financially support UNFPA, it needed to monitor what the Fund was doing in China. Given that the Senator's vote was essential to the government continuing to hold office, the necessary AusAID funds were found and the appointment made. As it happened, the staff member proved to be a very valuable addition to the office.

The remaining staff were all local appointees assigned by our counterpart Ministry for Foreign Trade and Economic Cooperation (MOFTEC). While they covered most of the administrative and financial work they also assumed key project responsibilities. Each had a personal story to recount. The older members told how they were sent to the countryside during the Cultural Revolution, the younger ones describing how they came from a provincial capital to study English in Beijing. Given that it was the nineties, none of the local staff ever invited us into their Chinese home as it was not officially encouraged to have personal contacts with foreigners. Was it perceived embarrassment at the status of their dwellings or did it have to do with the almost certain reporting of a visiting foreigner, a 'laowai', by a prying neighbour? Nonetheless, we enjoyed amicable relationships with all our colleagues and their families.

As with earlier assignments, a pattern began to emerge. Our children were enrolled in the International School (IBS), our apartment furnished, a car and "flying pigeon"[5] bicycles purchased, my wife found a job in AusAID located at the Australian Embassy, gym membership was secured, newspaper subscriptions placed and the World Service of the BBC located on my radio. These were positive steps yet I felt unsettled. I missed the atmosphere of Ghana, much to the surprise of my Chinese colleagues who assumed I would be pleased to be out of the African continent. I missed the space, speaking in English, the Ghanaian culture and, loathe as I was to admit it, the shared colonial heritage. China felt very foreign.

---

[5]Despite the speed implied in their name, these bikes were, in fact, made of cast iron, were very heavy and had no gears.

Soon came the Beijing winter. Early one brisk morning I stepped out of our apartment building wearing my smart leather shoes. As I slid on the ice, I only just managed to hang on without breaking a bone. Lesson one: wear rubber-soled shoes. Then, as I sat down in our office car where the engine had been running to pump out the heat, I was overwhelmed by the smell of cigarette smoke and garlic. I gagged but said nothing. Lesson two: get over it, especially since my driver was such a gentle and obliging man. I was also made uneasy when I became aware that my colleagues in New York HQ were observing and commenting on my performance. Unlike Ghana, where I only heard once from the African Director, China was of direct concern to the Executive Director. How senior management made its decisions about the Chinese programme was also something of a mystery. "They're meeting again", the desk officer at HQ would tell me. "What's going on?" I would ask her. "If I hear anything, I'll let you know". I certainly didn't know nor did she. We were not always in the loop. We were both very naive about the intricacies of internal politics.

In retrospect I should have questioned the lack of substantive briefing about our Chinese programme. Other than a note from my predecessor, the concerned geographic division provided no documents, no reading list and no suggested contacts.[6] Very likely, because I had never received any briefings prior to earlier postings, I just assumed this to be the norm. Over time I realized this lack of information had to do with the opaque way UNFPA headquarters dealt with the challenges presented by the Chinese family planning programme. China was a challenge for our Executive Committee insofar it felt bound to consider conflicting points of view and their impact on the respective domestic politics of a number of the Fund's key donors. For HQ it was the European capitals and Washington that mattered, not feedback from the country office in Beijing.

Being relatively new to the organisation and having never worked at headquarters, I lacked the HQ "connections" that would allow me to informally monitor what was going on. While I anticipated the Chinese would keep the administration of family planning a closely guarded secret I did not expect my exclusion from key decisions within my own organisation. For example, I found myself asking who were the decision-makers about China at headquarters? What were their objectives? Did they have any? Who prepared the

---

[6]Material available at that time included a Population Council paper published in *Population and Development Review*, Vol. 15, No 1 (Mar. 1989), titled "The United States, China, and the United Nations Population Fund: Dynamics of UN Policymaking". As an introductory reader this would have been very helpful but was only found by me years later. So much for a substantive briefing on what was UNFPA's biggest programme at the time and its most controversial!

briefing papers? What was said at strategy meetings? On what basis were decisions made? Who actually held the ball in this ideological game? I presumed my superiors in New York had the answers. What seemed to be at stake was how the UNFPA Executive Director made **her** decisions. In brief, what was happening in China was relevant only to the extent it affected the political battles being fought over abortion, and the US/China relationship. The intensified Chinese family planning strategy implemented in the two years prior to my arrival was a case in point.

In early 1991, following direction from party elders and the Central Committee and the State Council, the State Family Planning Commission (SFPC) under the guidance of the "Birth Planning Leading Group"[7] introduced the "responsibility system" for meeting FP targets. Officials from the provincial down to the village levels were warned that if their unit of responsibility recorded too many births, "...they would be held personally accountable". The consequences for the 900 million peasants from the resulting crackdown was "...enormous. In 1992, the total fertility rate fell to 1.86. This was the first time it had ever dropped below two births per couple. China had reached targets it had not expected to meet until 2010."[8] How this was achieved was the subject of enormous controversy. For UNFPA, following the publication of the Kristof article and other harsh criticisms of the coercive nature of the Chinese family planning programme, it was a major crisis. There were two sides to this. On one side, namely the European and the Australian, the Fund was recognised as the only significant donor working with the Chinese to ameliorate the worst aspects of the policy. Apart from the Ford and Rockefeller Foundations, there were no other international organisations working on family planning in China.

Despite global debates on the issues, no donor was prepared to pay the political cost. Consequently, UNFPA was seen as the most important conduit for information and influence.[9] We were the only game in town. Our programme was viewed internationally as having the potential to move the Chinese family planning effort towards something less harsh: to moving it away from its 'administrative' constraints whereby couples were told how many children they could have, when they could have them, all with the

---

[7]Susan Greenhalgh, JUST ONE CHILD SCIENCE AND POLICY IN DENG'S CHINA, University of California Press, Berkeley p. 22, 2008.

[8]Nicholas D. Kristof and Sheryl Wudunn, CHINA WAKES THE STRUGGLE FOR THE SOUL OF A RISING POWER, Times Books, New York, 1994, p. 236.

[9]The UNFPA programme began in China in 1979, although it was preceded by some limited activities. Since 1979 there had been three cycles of UNFPA support up to and including the period of my appointment, 1993–98 (CP1, 1980–1984 inclusive of support to the 1982 census and CP2, 1985–1989, each for $50 million and involving 64 projects then CP3, 1990–1994 for $57 million which continued many of the same projects but shifted some focus from urban to rural). All were fully implemented which is not always the case with UN assistance. Programmes are often underspent.

prospect of punishment if they did not adhere to this regime. The Republican Administration of the USA and its pro-life supporters around the world, including some members of the Australian parliament, seemed to believe (somewhat unfairly) that UNFPA was in some way complicit with the abuses. This belief persisted despite UNFPA's public opposition to China's conduct of its family planning programme particularly where it was found to be monitoring women's periods, aborting babies in the third trimester,[10] burning the house of couples who had a child out of 'quota', and taking away a couple's right to decide how many children they could have and when. So much was UNFPA linked with the Chinese programme that despite being repeatedly cleared by USAID of any involvement in coercion, and restrictions placed on any assistance going for abortions by its governing council,[11] presidents Reagan and George H. W, Bush cut their funding to UNFPA.[12] For example, in 1985, the US withheld $10 million of its $46 million contribution to the Fund, and from 1986 to 1992, it withdrew all funding. As the amounts were nearly 25% of the Fund's total income, this decision was of the utmost importance. But, as I was to discover, American support for UNFPA bounced between Democrat 'in' and Republican 'out'. On 22 January 1993, the newly elected President, Bill Clinton, signed an executive memorandum overruling the Republican policy and restored funding to UNFPA.[13] And, so it remained until George W. Bush was elected and swung the pendulum the other way redirecting the funds to USAID.[14]

Although largely driven by internal US politics, central to this public debate was UNFPA's presence in China and, by association, our link to their one-child policy and legalised abortion. Lacking any substantive briefing I could only learn by questioning my predecessor and piecing together what I learnt on the job. There was no paper trail. Thus began my first lesson into

---

[10]China has the highest number of abortions in the world, with an estimated 13 million performed annually. (Bethany Allen-Ebrahimian, "Meet China's Pro-Life Christians" Foreign Policy, August 5, 2015).

[11]UNFPA does not support abortion services but recognizes unsafe abortion as a major health problem. It seeks to reduce abortions and related deaths by improving access to contraception and to treatment for complications of unsafe abortion.

[12]In keeping with the Kemp-Kasten Amendment of 1985 to the appropriations bill and the "Mexico City policy" of 1984 denying funds to any non-governmental organisation that provided abortion counselling referral or services.

[13]But $10 m was withheld in view of UNFPA's assistance to the population programme in China and separate accounting was required.

[14]A pattern that continues to this day. Following the George W Bush cuts, President Obama restored funding only to have them cut by President Trump. Now, fulfilling promises made in his 2020 election campaign, President Biden restored US contributions to UNFPA on January 28, 2021. Secretary of State, Antony Blinken, said the State Department was "taking the necessary steps to make $32.5 million appropriated by Congress available in 2021 to support the United Nations Population Fund."

the Chinese programme and the way UNFPA dealt with it. As with earlier assignments, but to a greater extent in China, it was up to me to do the research.

In 1980, following the opening of its office in 1979, UNFPA's first Country Programme was instigated. Throughout the following decade the Fund helped China conduct a modern census, train demographers, and improve the quality of Chinese contraceptives thereby better protecting women's health and reducing the practice of unnecessary abortions. The $57 million five-year programme included 50 approved projects, mostly executed by specialist UN agencies. Of these, most had already concluded, such as an IUD study and a Norplant contraceptive trial. There were 11 pending projects including a so-called "model county project"—a $1 million project aimed at introducing internationally acceptable human rights[15] into selected counties. The intention here was to show that fertility reduction could be accomplished without coercion. The Chinese were very serious about our programme's assistance, and usually spent more than 95% of their matching financial allocation.

Timeline of UNFPA's presence in China.[16]

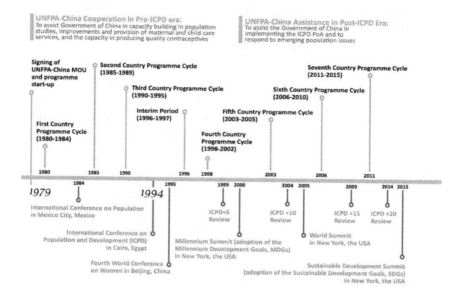

---

[15]Notwithstanding that the Chinese understanding of human rights is more of a collective concept as distinct from an individualistic favoured in the west. The gap in communication between Westerners and the Chinese is evident when the former talks about individual rights and demonises China for the lack of these and the Chinese talk about the rights of the community.

[16]UNFPA, UNFPA AND CHINA: 40 YEARS OF COOPERATION ON POPULATION AND DEVELOPMENT. UNFPA Country Office in China, 2019.

Throughout this period, there was also a patchwork of UN agencies which, despite some efforts to coordinate, led to much confusion and very little programme collaboration. The Chinese coordinating agency was known by its acronym, CICETE (China International Centre for Economic and Technical Exchanges). CICETE received 3% of its funding from UNDP and another 3% from implementing agencies as an execution fee.

The Chinese Department of International Trade and Economic Affairs (DITEA) of the Ministry of Foreign Trade and Economic Cooperation (MOFTEC) was UNFPA's coordinating agency. The staff there was generally very sincere about their work and committed to helping China. But when it came to using UNFPA funds to finance foreign consultants or paying for some of our experts coming from our Country Support Team (CST) based in Bangkok, they were very tough. They wanted every cent of the programme spent in China or on Chinese. They were also under a lot of pressure from other ministries which sometimes required them to take a strong stand. And when it came to political and policy questions, DITEA had no real authority. That rested with the State Family Planning Commission (SFPC).

The SFPC was UNFPA's chief counterpart. The Commission totally controlled policy, logistics, production, and contraceptive research and was led by the most powerful woman minister in China, Madame Peng Peiyun. Minister Peng was a member of the 11-person State Council, the top government entity at the time. Minister Peng was in charge of population, health, youth, and women's affairs. She was to be the focal point for the 1995 International Women's Conference in Beijing because of her oversight of the All China Women's Federation (ACWF). While SFPC was not one of the powerful "money makers" being separate from the more externally driven ministries, Madam Peng still had a lot of power. Having been appointed to the Ministry in 1988, she took over from what was said to be a lacklustre performance of a former moderate Minister. As the government's policy was comprehensively tightened under Peng's leadership, fertility dropped. Over time I came to know her story well.

Madam Peng was one of the most famous victims of the Cultural Revolution. One of the first to be paraded around Beijing wearing a dunce's hat, she later spent seven and a half years being "re-educated" on a vegetable farm. It must have been a bitter experience impacting on her most productive years. It was commonly said she was now making up for the lost time by working on her country's most important problem, population. Always polite and welcoming, she was nonetheless, tireless, smart and very formidable.[17] She was also said to be suspicious of 'laowai'.[18]

If this was the political context in which UNFPA was operating, how did the Chinese family planning programme (about which there was so much concern) actually work? Therein lay another challenge. To understand the context, I needed some history. The programme began in 1953. A long-awaited census in that year revealed that the population had reached 583 million, over 100 million more than the government expected. The consequence of this boom was heated debate over what was the best way to deal with the revelation. Chairman Mao believed it was capitalism, not overpopulation, that created widespread impoverishment. Believing that large families were the best way to build a strong nation, Mao encouraged more women to have babies.[19] The majority agreed with him. Consequently, China did not immediately recognise the significance of the population threat. The reassessment came following the millions of people who starved to death during the Great Leap forward between 1958 and 1961. When the 1964 census revealed that birth rates had again resumed high levels of growth which continued through the 1970's, lower birth quotas were implemented in the hope it would stabilise growth.[20] After this, the decision was made to establish a birth control office and campaigns were begun to promote late marriage and the two-child family. This, despite peasant resistance and opposition by health workers to include birth control among their services.[21]

In 1971, within the scope of a socialist planned economy, Premier Zhou Enlai instigated the 'birth planning' programme. Through rigorous campaigns, promoting the slogan "*wan, xi, shao*" (later, longer, fewer), people were asked to marry later, delay the first birth, and have fewer births. Regular visits to these women were made by health staff, midwives, barefoot doctors and FP workers and volunteers and they supplied the contraceptives and

---

[17]At that time, her husband was a newly elected member of the Politburo and her father was in Deng's inner circle, euphemistically, called the Sitting Committee. Even though that committee had no official standing, it effectively ran China.

[18]"*Laowai*" (老外) a common term for foreigners.

[19]For further details see Jonathan Watts, WHEN A BILLION CHINESE JUMP, (Faber and Faber, 2010), pp. 202–203.

[20]H. Yuan Tian, Zhang Tianlu, Ping Lu, Li Jingneng, Liang Zhongtang, China's Demographic Dilemmas, Population Bulletin, 1992, pp. 10–11.

[21]Jonathan Fenby, HISTORY OF MODERN CHINA: THE FALL AND RISE OF A GREAT POWER, Penguin.

referred clients to the state-run hospitals, government clinics and factory first aid centres for more permanent "devices" (i.e. IUD's).[22]

Although the programme was a success, the government decided it was not enough. In 1979 the State Council introduced a stringent family planning programme. At the time there were several theories about why the now commonly, but somewhat misleadingly known 'one-child policy', was introduced.[23] The first was linked to the advent of Deng's economic reforms in 1979 in which farmers were allowed to "privatise" excess produce after their allocated state quotas had been met. This created an incentive for farmers to have more children to work the land. The one child policy was intended to counteract that impulse. Another theory was that in order to limit total population to 1.2 billion by 2000, a new policy needed to be adopted that would radically restricted births. Yet another theory held that planning families was no different from other "state planning" in a socialist system. This last theory coincided with China's cultural mores which valued community well-being over individual rights. Whatever the reason, fertility dropped from almost six in the 1950s to around three at the start of the 1980s.[24] This one child/one couple decision was renewed in March 1995 by China's President Jiang Zemin. Family planning (FP) had become a 'fundamental' state policy.

The programme was a phenomenal success but how it was achieved was the subject of enormous controversy. The "responsibility system" introduced in 1991 saw provincial governors and party secretaries held personally accountable for meeting family planning targets. The consequences for 900 million peasants, three quarters of China's 1.2 billion population, "were enormous".[25] For the first time in Chinese history, the total fertility rate[26] had dropped to 1.86, and this had been achieved within two decades of launching the FP programme! "It would be difficult to imagine any policy anywhere in the world having such a huge effect on the daily lives of so many people".[27]

---

[22]Susan Greenhalgh and Edwin A. Winckler, GOVERNING CHINA'S POPULATION: FROM LENINIST TO NEOLIBERAL BIOPOLITICS (Stanford University Press, 2005), pp. 85–87.

[23]For further details see Jonathan Watts, op cit pp. 204.

[24]H. Yuan Tian, Zhang Tianlu, Ping Lu, Li Jingneng, Liang Zhongtang, *China's Demographic Dilemmas*, Population Bulletin, 1992, pp. 14–15.

[25]Nicholas D. Kristof, Sheryl Wudunn, CHINA WAKES: THE STRUGGLE FOR THE SOUL OF A RISING POWER, Times Books, 1994, New York. p. 236.

[26]"The average number of children that would be born per woman if all women lived to the end of their childbearing years and bore children according to a given fertility rate at each age. A rate of two children per woman is considered the replacement rate for a population, resulting in relative stability in terms of total numbers". C.I.A, 'World Factbook', Accessed 6 November 2017, https://www.cia.gov/library/publications/the-world-factbook/docs/notesanddefs.html?countryName=France&countryCode=fr&regionCode=eu#2127.

[27]Nicholas D. Kristof, Sheryl Wudunn, op cit, p. 236.

The population growth rate when I arrived in 1993 was now roughly equal to that of the United States, a country equal in size to China but far more habitable given that the western half of China is relatively dry and barren. So how did they do it? Given my limited briefing from head office, plus the little I had gleaned from general sources or heard from my predecessor, I had very little idea. Added to this, when I arrived, the actual population control methods employed were a closely guarded secret. Unlike today, provincial FP guidelines were neither in English nor on the internet. They were very difficult to obtain, especially for a foreigner.

The overall policy was decided centrally in Beijing with implementation determined at provincial level. Whilst there were variations from province to province, the strategy was basically the same. If you were a Han Chinese couple born in a city you could apply to the appropriate official for a 'quota' to have a child in your fourth year of marriage—the policy being to delay marriage and births. If permission was given and there was a successful delivery, irrespective of the sex of the child, no more children were permitted. An intrauterine device (IUD) was then inserted and when the child was approximately ten years of age, female sterilization was encouraged.

If you were a Han farmer and your place of household registration (your 'hukou') was rural and your first child at four years was a girl, you could apply for a second 'quota' at eight years in the hope that this time you would have a boy. Irrespective of the sex of the child who might then be born, the same regimen of contraception would be applicable as with the one child, only now were you restricted to two. If you were of non-Han origin (belonging to a 'minority ethnic group'), you were permitted to have three children with the same birth spacing only this time spread over 12 years. Should a pregnancy occur out of 'quota', that is, without permission, abortion was recommended. When this was ignored, and an 'infringement' occurred whereby the couple insisted on going to term, a mix of penalties was incurred. These could consist of fines, confiscation of produce, loss of seniority, withdrawal of scholarships, demotion at the workplace, public shaming, withdrawal of party membership and being dropped off the priority housing list.

At the time of my arrival, 27 provinces and three cities had family planning regulations based on the national policy. Seen as particularly onerous were the Sichuan regulations then viewed as the benchmark for the 13 or so provinces that did not have any regulations but were considering drafting them. It is important to note that it was the provincial regulations applicable to your ethnicity and your place of birth that determined the number of children you were permitted to have, irrespective of where you might move to live later in life: be it to Beijing as a Ph.D. student or Shanghai as a builder's labourer or Lhasa as a provincial official.

More reported on than the harshness of the regulations were the alleged violations of human rights accompanying them. In the first instance these were the routine monitoring of people's, mostly women's, reproductive lives: the checking on their fertility cycles and any delays to it. In the second were the 'unofficial' measures whereby 'persuasion' by the official methods was not successful. These gave rise to international protests over the alleged sanctioned sterilisation of the mentally ill, coercion of ethnic Tibetans, substantial property seizures, the burning of homes, abduction of relatives, and the handcuffing of pregnant women.[28] There were also concerns raised about the very high sex ratio that suggested either underreporting of girl births in order to try for a boy, infanticide or sex-selective abortion. Officials who had recorded a poor performance in meeting family planning quotas were now compelled by a "responsibility system" to meet their quotas, by whatever means. These included sterilisations, an over reliance on the unreliable and late-term abortions, despite the availability of the full range of modern contraceptives.

The Chinese always maintained there were bound to be overzealous officials at local levels in such a huge programme and that these cadres were disciplined when they used unsatisfactory methods that contravened the regulations. They would have preferred not to have such a policy, they said, insisting that a couple could have as many children as they wanted as long as they had sufficient funds and were willing to pay. The government argued the policy was necessary, given China's population size and the need to lift millions out of poverty. Any couple having additional children beyond their 'quota' meant they were inflicting a cost on a poor and developing country. In the Party's view, such social irresponsibly could not be ignored. The offending couple had to pay a "social compensation fee" for the extra numbers.[29] The dilemma was crudely put by a rhetorical statement I heard time and time again: "What is it you want? Boatloads of starving Chinese sailing up the Hudson into New York or a prosperous China, caring for its people?"[30]

---

[28]'Forced abortion and sterilization in china: the view from the inside hearing before the subcommittee on international operations and human rights of the committee on international relations house of representatives one hundred fifth congress second session', June 10, 1998, http://commdocs. house.gov/committees/intlrel/hfa49740.000/hfa49740_0f.htm.

[29]The "black children" as they are sometimes referred to (The Economist, August 21, 2010).

[30]There are now more than 1.4 billion people in China. The Government has consistently maintained that the figure would be 1.7 billion had it not initiated the programme. Clifford Coonan, "*Chinese family fear for father after horror of forced abortion*" The Independent, 27 June 2012.

The cost of executing this policy was huge. More than 500,000 people worked directly in the area and many of the fines or property confiscations provided revenue that sustained this bureaucracy.[31] Over and above this number, there were millions and millions of staff, directly or indirectly, running campaigns and then routinely monitoring people's reproductive lives to either punish or reward.[32] In financial terms, the administrative costs were enormous.

For me, three things brought the controversy surrounding the programme into stark relief. First, the ongoing firestorm of criticism associated with the implementation of Chinese policy. Understandably, claims of abuse arising from this policy represented an easy target for conservative US governments and Vatican based anti-abortion forces. China's methods were increasingly under the scrutiny of international observers and UNFPA was engaged in continuous dialogues with interested parties.[33]

Second, the 1990 census in China produced the same fertility rate of 2.3 as recorded in 1982, thus prompting the "re-politicisation" of the programme. Chinese planners were doubly alarmed when they saw the large reproductive cohort resulting from unchecked births during the early years of the Cultural Revolution.

Third, in 1991, political and party leaders at all levels were made accountable for meeting population targets. While the so-called "responsibility system" was not a directly coercive policy, it created a climate for abuse. People were viewed not as humans but as statistical goals. It led to what appeared to be significant increases in coercion including massive sterilisation, destruction of private property and extreme financial penalties. China's Family Planning Association[34] became the local party enforcer of this new policy, while at the same time lobbying for better health care.

In 1992 a SFPC fertility survey was followed by an SFPC press conference announcing dramatic reductions in births and fertility, prompting UNFPA to increase pressure on the Chinese government to moderate its policies or risk losing UNFPA assistance. Letters were written by the Executive Director to

---

[31]The Australian, September 17, 2010.

[32]Information Office of the State Council Of the People's Republic of China, Family Planning in China, (August 1995, Beijing), http://www.china-un.ch/eng/bjzl/t176938.htm.

[33]Barbara B. Crane and Jason L. Finkle, *The United States, China, and the United Nations Population Fund: Dynamics of US Policymaking*, Population and Development Review, Vol. 15, No. 1 (Mar. 1989), pp. 23–59 http://www.jstor.org/stable/1973404 Accessed: 02-09-2017 08:58 UTC.

[34]"All 30 provinces, autonomous regions and centrally administered municipalities as well as the overwhelming majority of the cities, counties and grass-roots units have set up their family planning associations, totalling more than one million with approximately 80 million members. Their members keep in close touch with the broad masses of the couples of childbearing age." Information Office of the State Council Of the People's Republic of China, op cit, p. 6.

the Foreign Minister, and the SFPC Minister, expressing the Fund's concern and demanding answers. The Kristof article in the New York Times exposed the crisis and led to UNFPA sending a team of demographers to review the 1992 data. The team comprised internationally renowned demographers with a brief to examine why the Chinese birth rate had fallen so dramatically (below replacement level) in the previous decade. In Susan Greenhalgh and Edwin Winckler's book (2005) they explained how five years of family planning campaigns up to the 1992 had dramatic and unsustainable effects on China's birth rate. As well as pushing China's birth rate below replacement levels, the birth policy also strained relations between party cadres and the people. In their view, this gave China enough incentive to gradually move towards new and less rigid guidelines for family planning.[35]

However, UNFPA'S critics didn't see it this way. US Republican, Chris Smith from New Jersey,[36]Australian Senator Brian Harradine, and conservative members of the British House of Commons, routinely condemned UNFPA for being in China.[37] They declared our presence to be an affirmation of a FP programme that was coercive, contrary to basic human rights and only sustained through forced abortions and sterilizations. But this was not the case. UNFPA did not support China's FP methods. We sought to find more humane ways for people to exercise choice. We did so by offering dialogue and support to reproductive health services that were based on providing complete information, choices of contraceptives, informed decisions, guidance and counselling for women.

Against this background, my colleagues and I sat down in 1994 to negotiate with the government the Fourth UNFPA Country Programme of Assistance to China. Two years later we reached agreement. Along the way there were multiple challenges not least of which was that we never thought it would take so long.

---

[35]Greenhalgh, S, Winckler, E.A, GOVERNING CHINA'S POPULATION: FROM LENINIST TO NEOLIBERAL BIOPOLITICS, Stanford California, Stanford University Press, 2005, p. 134.

[36]At the time of writing, Chris Smith was senior a member on the Foreign Affairs Committee and Chairman of the Africa, Global Health, Global Human Rights and International Organization Subcommittee.

[37]Allegations about UNFPA activities in China gathered by the Population Research Institute, a non-profit U.S. research group, seems to have been instrumental in persuading US President George W. Bush not to sign over $34 m which had been earmarked for the UN Population Fund in 2001. Greg Barrow, 'Abortion row threatens UN funds', BBC, Wednesday, 27 February 2002, http://news.bbc.co.uk/2/hi/americas/1843208.stm.

Much has now been written on negotiating with the Chinese. In 1994 the most pertinent advice I received came from the New Zealand ambassador who was a student of Chinese history. He quoted "Chinese Gordon"[38], a British army officer and administrator who, in 1860, served in China during the Second Opium War and the Taiping Rebellion. He was said to have concluded, once you had reached your negotiated position, that you should stick to it and simply repeat it, always courteously, again and again. I adopted this practice although, despite repetition, I did not always know how UNFPA's position was being received nor on what basis our counterparts made their decisions.

I soon came to realise that the Chinese had different perspectives on many levels: history, past glories, humiliations, and recent achievements. Greatly appreciated were foreign partners who were knowledgeable about Chinese culture as well as those who tried to speak Mandarin. At a superficial level, I was also aware of the behavioural 'do's and don'ts' as applied to westerners living in the country. But I needed to remember I was negotiating with government counterparts not doing a business deal. In this context, I could never forget that my counterparts were communist party members and that in my own office there were also party members.[39] I assumed our phones would be tapped, if the occasion demanded, as was reported to be common practice in the eighties.[40] E-mail was the least secure means of communication.

Throughout the negotiation process I gained valuable insight into the importance of the UN to the Chinese government as well as to the associated think tanks with which I interacted. While the amount of money UNFPA provided was negligible, our presence in the country gave the entities charged with delivering the FP programme some legitimacy. With that came the responsibility for delivering projects and managing the assigned funding. The public servants involved, whatever their motivation, stood to benefit. Our funding facilitated their attendance at international training courses, study tours, equipment upgrades, and provincial travel on the higher UN daily allowance. We traded on these practices because it gave us a strong bargaining tool with which to negotiate change.

---

[38]Following the death in 1885 of Major General Gordon at Khartoum in the Sudan, 100,000 Melbourne citizens contributed to a statue which was erected in 1889 and can be seen in the Gordon Reserve, Spring Street, Melbourne, near to Parliament House.

[39]One of our minor successes when dealing with the government was to insist they gave us a choice when filling vacancies in our office. Previously, the counterpart ministry to UNFPA, MOFTEC, would simply delegate a staff member to the office but we insisted that at least we be given a list of names for interview and ultimate selection and appointment. This, somewhat reluctantly, was finally agreed to.

[40]New York Times, May 15, 1993.

As UNFPA was a solitary player, our views on the process of the negotiations were eagerly sought by all the diplomatic missions monitoring the Chinese human rights situation.[41] While the embassies didn't want to be involved, too sensitive a topic for them, they wanted to be kept informed. One way of doing this was to regularly organise field trips to the provinces for interested ambassadors. The first of many such trips was in March 1994 to Gansu and Ningxia with the ambassadors of Sweden, Norway, Denmark, and the First Secretary of Finnish Embassy. When we travelled to the provinces, even though we were always accompanied by government counterparts, we had, surprisingly, access to whatever was of interest and to whomever would answer questions. Proudly villagers, factory workers and commune officials would tell us how rigorously they were enforcing government policies unaware of the controversial elements that should have been avoided. It was the official line being passed down from the top and repeated over and over at every level of government.

Were the set numerical targets for contraceptive use, and the ceiling on birth 'quotas' always achieved by a province or city? I was never sure. Certainly the concerned official told me they were seeing them as mandatory requirements by which their performance would be measured. In the absence of anything else, (e.g. quality of care, contraceptive choice) it was all they knew. But there were those among my ministerial counterparts who were aware of the bigger issues. As we travelled together or socialised at a banquet they would vigorously defend the policy while acknowledging there was substantial room for improvement in its delivery.

What this taught me was the importance of sitting down quietly with our Chinese counterparts and discussing how the government programme could better comply with a voluntary approach to family planning. Towards this goal, I established a working group of various UN organisations to discuss how best to integrate international standards of women's reproductive rights and quality of care. From our regular dialogues with SFPC we knew they were willing to adopt new methods, including a more user-oriented approach, provided government goals were maintained. This was valuable leverage that helped to achieve some international standards.

During the negotiations neither party was in a hurry. The Chinese took their time, they avoided risks and referred anything controversial to a higher authority. For our part we wanted to make sure we were looking after our UN mandate and maintaining the confidence of international donors. We met our

---

[41]Building on this we would periodically arrange rural inspection tours by interested ambassadors.

counterparts at either the UNFPA office or at the foreign relations departments of the concerned ministries. We knew it was never going to be easy, made more so because one never knew quite what was going on. Throughout the two years of meetings the government pendulum swung between rigid adherence and relaxation; between policy enforcers and demographers who were monitoring the data; and between the bureaucrats in the departments and the progressives in the think tanks.

Key to adhering to our mandate and critical, as we saw it, to the future of the Chinese FP programme was improving the status of women, particularly in the rural areas. The Minister assured us that all the grassroots activities of the "All China Women's Federation (ACWF)" would now be directed at improving women's status, while reducing fertility. Although this reinforced gender stereotypes, it was a step in the right direction. Obviously, you weren't going to immediately change centuries old patriarchal traditions. People had always wanted a son to pass on the family line. Typically, the husband and his mother dominated this decision in which the future mother-to-be had no part. When we identified this problem, we launched a campaign to counter this view while at the same time improving the quality of services to ensure survival. Maternal and infant mortality were still far too high, especially among ethnic minorities and remote communities. This was not the showcase capital, Beijing, we were talking about.

What we could not change but sought to highlight was the bureaucratic rivalry between the Ministry of Public Health (MOPH) and SFPC. The former traced its history back to the founding of the republic while the latter was a well-funded newcomer. Employing half a million workers with a clear mandate to control population growth, the Commission was still depended on MOPH to deliver the clinical services. There was some integration at a senior level with the same minister in charge of both ministries and relevant vice-ministerial discussions before joint statements were issued. But SFPC service centres continued to expand, even adjacent to a government health clinic, and they took to including MCH among their responsibilities. This was not the integration of family planning and reproductive health we hoped for.

A crucial change to the political environment surrounding the China programme was the International Conference on Population and Development (ICPD) held in Cairo in September 1994. This was a special conference, a "quantum leap" as one author called it[42] because it marked

---

[42] Stanley Johnson THE POLITICS OF POPULATION: CAIRO 1994 (Earthscan, London, 1995), p. 9.

a shift from a national approach governed by numbers to one measured by individual human rights. 179 countries adopted the Programme of Action (POA) at Cairo one of whose principles[43] stated:

> Reproductive health-care programmes should provide the widest range of services without any form of coercion. All couples and individuals have the basic right to decide freely and responsibly the number and spacing of their children and to have the information, education and means to do so.[44]

This principle declared that the decision to have children, when and how many, was none of the state's business. It was for individuals and couples to decide! This ICPD POA principle was reinforced in September 1995, by the Platform for Action of the Fourth World Conference on Women held in Beijing when it affirmed:

> The human rights of women include their right to have control over and decide freely and responsibly on matters related to their sexuality, including sexual and reproductive health, free of coercion, discrimination and violence[45]

So how did the Chinese navigate around these international agreements or more to the point, how did UNFPA? Let's deal with the UNFPA first. Every international agreement, of necessity, obtains clauses which reinforce national sovereignty otherwise countries would never agree to them. The ICPD POA was no exception. The opening paragraph to the principles adopted in Cairo declared

> The implementation of the recommendations contained in the programme of action is the sovereign right of each country, consistent with national laws and development priorities...[46]

This insistence on sovereignty was reinforced by Dr. Sadik in her concluding statement.

---

[43] Note that the approach adopted in Cairo was a holistic one emphasising poverty, women's status, and the structure of society and that it was only agreed to following compromises over issues of adolescent sexuality, unsafe abortion and sexual rights. In fact, so controversial were these subjects that the divisions opened up have seen no global conferences on population and reproductive health held ever since: the fear being that the POA could be wound back.

[44] Principle 8, Programme of Action adopted at the International Conference on Population and Development, Cairo, 5–13 September 1994.

[45] Notes, State of World Population 1997, UNFPA.

[46] Programme of Action, ICPD, Chapter ii, 'Principles', Cairo, September 1994, P. 8.

Nothing in the Programme of Action limits the freedom of nations to act individually within the bounds of their laws and cultures...[47]

With these standard caveats, China was able to declare the ICPD a "Landmark triumph in the history of the international cause of population and family planning..." and that the POA contained, "...the guiding principles for population and family planning programmes for the entire world".[48] It was a "delicate consensus", we were later told by the Chinese in a meeting with SFPC, thereby reinforcing Peng Peiyun's speech at Cairo in which she declared that China had

> ...been adhering to the principle of combining government guidance and voluntariness of the people.[49]

Given this agreement, the ICPD POA was one document that everyone could, for the most part, act upon. The Programme had put population into a development process whereby responses to the needs of individuals mattered rather than demographic goals. By so doing FP programmes had broadened into reproductive health, improving the quality of care and opposition to state incentives and disincentives.[50]

On this basis, I now included in our negotiations in Beijing questions about how the ICPD was going to be implemented; and how the POA was to be interpreted by the interested parties. Of course, complications arose. Some of the Chinese specialists believed the goal of voluntarism should be accompanied by government guidance. This was flexibility without publicity. Others felt a "remarkable lack of transparency on the part of UNFPA".[51] They felt they had been "done in" by the international community. Some ambassadors I spoke with argued that China should not be given concessions regarding the ICPD's already agreed upon wording. I felt we needed to push the authorities into removing the "administrative controls" (targets and quotas). But there was no way China would openly admit the quota

---

[47]"The principle of sovereignty underlies the whole text. Nothing...can or should be interpreted as interfering in any way with the nation's sovereign right to make and carry out policy according to its own laws, precepts, culture, and moral codes. That is fundamental, and dates from the earliest days of discussion on population. It is, in fact, the principle that makes all international discussion on population possible." Dr. Sadik quoted in Stanley Johnson, op cit, p. 98. Also see p. 204.

[48]Madam Peng Peiyun, op cit, p. 1.

[49]Stanley Johnson, Op cit, p. 198.

[50]Ian Howie, Notebook 4, pp. 1–2.

[51]Notebook 4, Dr. Huang, p. 7.

system needed to change. As a consequence, UNFPA projects could only be introduced in counties where there was less stringent family planning.[52]

Added to the complexity were some untimely developments that weighed heavily on the programme's success. When the Chinese delegation returned from Cairo, they were shocked to discover that a new Vice Minister had been appointed in their absence. He was there waiting for them. Why had he been appointed? they asked. There were clearly internal divisions within the Commission over how far the family planning programme should be moving. Mme Peng Peiyun was looking for a service-oriented programme, but in her efforts to explain what this meant, she was not well understood by her comrades, so the emphasis on targets and quotas held out. Meanwhile, at the provincial level, deputy governors responsible for population matters were never exposed to the debate, leaving such matters to the provincial party leader and the provincial director of the family planning programme. Their advancement depended on how well or otherwise they achieved their allocated quotas and targets.

Given these challenges, the future evolvement of the FP programme was difficult to resolve. Modifications were welcomed but cautiously introduced. Nonetheless, there were progressives in the government who could see the benefits of softening the existing FP policies. Their proposals were scheduled to be discussed later during the annual meeting of the Politburo in the spring of 1995. Clearly, it was important to us that we influence the outcome of this debate and move it towards the ICPD goals.[53] We wanted to demonstrate there were alternatives to their designated path.[54]

Following a key Vice Minister's visit to the Philippines on a UNFPA fellowship, he understood better the impact economics had on women's desire to have fewer children. Although proof of good practices elsewhere was never going to be enough in itself, we hoped this would be the message conveyed to the leaders at the annual meeting.

Evidence suggests that the modifications sought came later at a meeting on population statistics with representatives from the provinces. There, a much respected academic[55] expressed the view that a 'balancing act' was needed in

---

[52] Notebook 4, p.8.

[53] Notebook 4, p. 10.

[54] Notebook 4, p. 23.

[55] Dr. Gu Baochang was the Deputy Director of the Chinese Population Information and Research Centre from 1990 to 1998. He previously worked for UNFPA from 1988 to 1989 as a development adviser. Dr. Gu is still a prominent researcher on demographics and is currently located at the Centre for Population and Development Studies Renmin University of China, Beijing. https://baike.baidu.com/item/顾宝昌.

China. On one side he said, the administered programme, if tightened-up, would scare people. Under-reporting would then lead to greater corruption. On the other side, he continued, more and more people realised China had to change, but with quotas not yet eliminated, change could only come slowly. Every step we moved, he said, meant we would be continually looking over our shoulder. As one moved forward, there would always be others that would resist change. From this summary, I realised how delicate the situation was and how easily officials who questioned the system, could be isolated. It was going to take time to convince senior ministers to change their views, especially the single-minded stalwarts. Patience, particularly at province level, was the only way to proceed. Such was the political environment, we had to talk about what we were doing together rather than our differences.[56]

From headquarters, we heard that Dr. Sadik recognised what the Communists had done to change the status of women, but she felt progress could have been much better. China's targets and quotas were continuing to spark international discussion, but despite their commitment to ICPD, Sadik wanted to hear how the Chinese believed change could happen. UNFPA's Executive Board had also asked exactly what the role of UNFPA would be post-Cairo. It was reported that there were a variety of views. Some said UNFPA should continue its traditional role, but with a stronger advocacy focus. Others thought it should have a broader role in reproductive health by attending to all services. My own view was that we should promote reproductive health at the grassroots level.

In response to Sadik's statements, the Minister for MOFTEC[57] relayed the message that while the Chinese government attached great importance to its relationship with UNFPA, the policy could not be amended just because the international community wanted it. This was not to say UNFPA was merely a symbolic presence, the Fund was valued because of the expertise it brought. "In the last decade, you have given us $10 million a year to help the development of China", the Minister declared adding how the population policies of China had made a great contribution to lowering global population levels. But then, when explaining how China was experimenting with a market economy, he pointed out how approaches towards family planning

---

[56] Notebook 4, p. 23.

[57] Long Yongtu was also a diplomat based in New York before taking the reins at MOFTEC http://www.chinavitae.com/biography/Long_Yongtu, https://www.bloomberg.com/research/stocks/people/person.asp?personId=8214294&capId=115573972&previousCapId=115573972&previousTitle=GOODBABY%20INTERNATIONAL%20HOLDI, http://www.china.org.cn/business/Boao_Forum_2012/2012-03/31/content_25037464.htm.

were no different. He used the words 'laboratory' and 'transition', which we interpreted as a willingness to adapt to new circumstances.[58]

These comments of the Minister highlighted the crucial role UNFPA was playing in broadening the discussion within China's family planning bureaucracy. As the only agency able to negotiate at this level, it reinforced my belief that we needed to be there. Although our financial contribution was small relative to what the Chinese spent themselves, I saw how our programme exposed China to international issues beyond its borders, how it gave, for example, SFPC cadres a broader perspective beyond population statistics.

This was a theme Dr. Sadik took up with Mme Peng Peiyun at a meeting in February 1995 to discuss ICPD implementation. Dr. Sadik said how pleased she was to hear that China was improving reproductive health services and that population policies were being considered as more than just narrow demographic goals. In reply, Mme Peng explained how dealing with so many people meant it was impossible to manage without 'administrative controls'. She reiterated how in the 20 years of China's FP Programme, fertility had declined within a relatively stable political and economic climate. This presumed, she said, a strong underlying conviction that people supported the existing policies. If not, there would be a high chance of civil unrest.[59]

It was now becoming evident to us that the Chinese were seeking to strike a balance between the rights of individuals and the obligations of society. We knew that when it came to individual rights, we had to move delicately. Unlike the west, it was and is still common in China to view the family as the smallest nucleus rather than the individual. Feeding, clothing, and sheltering the family was seen as the most basic human right rather than individual choice free of state intervention. Thus, it was no good berating them for not meeting our moral standards. It would only be seen as unwarranted interference. Vice-Minister Dr. Peng Yu explained it this way. Take, for example, he said, the densely populated and underdeveloped province of Jiangsu, rigid adherence to the ICPD PoA would impose upon the authorities the need to choose between human rights or the overuse of resources. Choosing one or the other, he concluded, would have negative consequences.

To us, this example highlighted how ICPD's findings on reproductive health and its relationship to sustainable development was not widely understood in Beijing and if this was the case, it would be even less understood in the provinces. Quality of care and choice, both central to ICPD, would not have been in their frame of reference (nor, would it seem, in the Vice

---

[58]Notebook 4, p. 27–28.
[59]Notebook 4, p. 31–33.

Minister's). In principle, Mme Peng Peiyun did not object to there being no quotas, but she did insist there had to be some sense of cohesiveness. China did not want chaos.

So began a delicate unpublicised negotiation to produce a very carefully worded agreement. China insisted on maintaining its FP policies, and provinces their regulations, but within these limits we could negotiate an end to quotas and targets as well as insist on the enforcement of laws preventing coercion. We agreed that Peng Peiyun would lead this process through the education of cadres at SFPC and, via the Commission's outreach expose provincial leaders to the changes sought plus inform people of their choices when it came to family planning.[60]

Over time our meetings with our counterparts saw different priorities emerge. On the Chinese side, they sought to assure us they had studied the ICPD PoA and that the proposed country programme was within the ICPD framework. But both MOFTEC and the SFPC pushed for agreement on a standard text, consistent with other country programme documents, where no specific references were singled out for policy modifications. They preferred any experimentation to be implemented later. They said the existing FP programme needed to slow down first before any U-turn could be made. To suddenly announce there were to be no targets or quotas may lead to confusion and "who would take responsibility for that?" Abandoning now could see the situation get out of control. One of the main fears they cited, was that publicity may encourage people to migrate to other provinces where there were no quotas and targets. Stability and encouragement, not strangulation, were the key messages. "We want success. We want to improve our methods, but where is the justice if free choice means having a baby which cannot be fed, clothed or sheltered? We want improved living standards and women's education to lead to declining fertility. The policy as a whole cannot be changed!"

End of story? No. Cautious experimentation through careful preparation, education, and mobilisation but within the existing framework was acceptable, a compromise between social responsibility and the rights of individuals. Only then, if the programme were successful, could it be expanded. But above all, no publicity, with Mme Peng Peiyun reminding us she did not want to give the public the idea there was to be a relaxation in the overall policy.

---

[60]Notebook 4, p. 33–37.

As the negotiations wound on we were advised that it was important we reach agreement before SFPC reported to the State Council. If they reported now to Prime Minister Li Peng, he would resist any compromise reputedly having said, "we cannot make changes and if worse comes to worst we can do without UNFPA assistence". This was not just a face-saving exercise by the Chinese, it reflected the Chinese position whereby an international organisation could not give direction to a sovereign state. But what was an acceptable number of compromises they were prepared to make without appearing to lose ownership of a key government programme, and what were we prepared to accept? Our counterparts wanted to maintain ownership over their national initiatives, not just report that UNFPA insisted the Government make compromises.[61] For our side it was left up to me.

On the eve of Dr. Sadik's departure from China, following these high level meetings, we were informed that our request for an audience with President Jiang Zemin had been granted. President Jiang would meet us the following day at Zhongnanhai, the party headquarters located on the western side of the Forbidden City. On arrival, we were ushered into one of the formal reception rooms arranged in the traditional Chinese style. The President, along with his interpreter and senior government officials, sat to one side and Dr. Sadik and I, with our interpreter, on the other. Following the usual introductory pleasantries and the mandatory cups of tea, we gave an account of the progress we had made in our negotiations. The president listened, nodded, and smiled when he heard of the progress we had made. UNFPA may have been a footnote on his agenda, but it was clearly important for him that China maintained its profile within the UN system. Midway through the exchange and much to my horror, my mobile phone began ringing. I tried to switch it off pushing button after button. Phones were new to us at the time and we had hired them especially for Dr. Sadik's visit. It continued to ring. "Switch it off" hissed Dr. Sadik. I was mortified, until President Zhang leaned in and whispered to his interpreter, "Don't worry, it happens to all of us!"

In July of 1995, the UNRC met with Dr. Sadik in New York. He thought the Government was trying to 'muddle-through' in order to find a mutually acceptable compromise. "Nothing wrong with that" said Dr. Sadik. The Chinese then asked to talk to the Secretary-General about the problem. It was the UNRC's view that the Secretary-General, despite a briefing beforehand by Dr. Sadik, would be "rather accommodating" when it came to be dealing with the Chinese.[62] Back in Beijing things continued to move forward. By

---

[61] Notebook 5, p. 25–26.
[62] Notebook 5, p. 29.

September, it was reported to me that the Chinese appreciated the viewpoint of UNFPA and would come up with a project which incorporated the wishes of the Fund. For this, I resolved to reiterate our concerns to the authorities that "we would support you in the future regarding reproductive health activities, provided certain principles enshrined in the agreement reached were documented", namely, the basic ICPD principles covering volunteerism, an absence of coercion, contraceptive choice and routine monitoring of the project to ensure adherence. If the authorities agreed, a draft submission could be made. Time was limited. A new country programme would need to be written, discussed with the Chinese, edited, translated and be ready for the April 1996 meeting of the UNFPA Executive Board. This would mean a holding arrangement of at least 6 months between our current programme and any new one, but an indication by November that we were going to have a programme.[63]

The Three Integrations[64] Conference in the Sichuan capital, Chengdu, at the end of 1995, saw vice-governors, provincial ministers and representatives of various semi-organisations meet. The main aim was to clarify principles and commit to a new programme that would more effectively control population growth under the banner of economic growth. Mme Peng summarised the challenges facing China, reminding us that 70 million were still considered to be in poverty. Only last month, she said, China had adopted the "Agenda 21" document,[65] requiring the country take a comprehensive approach to solving population challenges. This meant it was not just numbers that mattered but the quality of education, health and social welfare. These were all connected to the status of women, their rights, and those of children, all earmarked as focus areas to managing China's FP situation. Consequently, FP workers needed to provide better services and coordinate their work but given the long years of focusing on childbearing, she concluded, this would take time. While there had been a decline in fertility during the 8th Five-year Plan (1991–1995)[66] through the "administrative" approach[67] this was not stable because the "fertility intentions of people had

---

[63]Notebook 5, p. 34–35.

[64]"Developing agricultural village economy; helping farmers achieve a modestly comfortable standard of living; and constructing "civilised and happy" families. These were seen by Peng Peiyun as a "road of hope" for rural family planning. Greenhalgh and Winckler op. cit. page 143.

[65]United Nations, Institutional aspects of sustainable development in China, Agenda 21, http://www.un.org/esa/agenda21/natlinfo/countr/china/inst.htm.
    Agenda 21, United Nations Conference on Environment & Development, https://sustainabledevelopment.un.org/content/documents/Agenda21.pdf.

[66]The 8th Five-Year Plan (1991–1995), http://www.china.org.cn/english/MATERIAL/157625.htm.

[67]During this period population growth rates reportedly dropped from 14.39% in 1990 to 10.55% in 1995. http://www.china.org.cn/english/MATERIAL/157625.htm.

not changed in a sustainable way". Farmers needed to understand the benefits of FP and cadres needed to better address the requirements of farmers.
Such an approach would generate more yuan, and by doing so help farmers
contribute to economic development.[68] Mme Peng also informed us that
some local FP workers felt their work was too difficult and that many were
tired and frustrated, especially when dealing with the 'unpredictable' floating
migrants. She said they needed to understand integration, to change their
management systems and adopt new working methods.

When we came to negotiating actual text in 1996, any agreement on the
Chinese side to even the most minor point granted to us, was seen by them
as a win to our side. Mind you, lacking little or no guidance from headquarters, it was left to us to decide what to give away or maintain. On and on
went the discussions. We debated back and forth and then we often agreed,
but by no means always, with the Chinese bottom line. They were, after all,
a sovereign state, managing the most populated country on earth and with
whom UNFPA had its largest programme. When approval was required for
changes to key sections of the document, my counterparts usually referred
them to more senior staff. This was not a problem as I had surprising access
to vice-ministerial and ministerial level officials, highlighting the importance
of our document. Ultimate approval, however, would come from Premier Li
Peng.[69]

What did help to clarify our position was when it was finally made clear
by Dr. Sadik that UNFPA was in China to stay. In a phone call she declared
that our programme would continue regardless of American domestic politics. What was important, she said, was "...not the different views between
SFPC, DIR and the MOH concerning coordination of projects—we were
not obligated to support their national programme nor did we agree with
it—what mattered were the international commitments made at Cairo. We
were operating in a global and UN environment". In reply Minister Long
Yongtu reminded me, "If there is no programme in China, UNFPA should
not be called a world body!". But rather than seeing this as a threat, I saw
the comparative advantage we had as a politically neutral international body.
They needed us, and we needed to keep it that way.

Thereafter, things changed, and notably so when we got down to talking
about money. The decision was made from headquarters that the amount of
money China was to receive was much less than before ($57 million down to

---

[68]Notebook 5, p. 42–43.
[69]"*Accomplishments of China's Family Planning Program's Family Planning Program: A Statement by a
Chinese Official.*" Population and Development Review 19, no. 2 (June 1993): 399. https://doi.org/
10.2307/2938455.

$20 million).[70] This became a real sticking point. During the negotiations, I had to adjust to being told that China was a poor, developing country. They saw this as an important reference point when the document would finally go before the UNFPA Executive Board. Whilst it was certainly true there were substantial areas of extreme poverty in the country, there was also abundant evidence of very rapid development. Adding to my doubts about this line of argument was concern about whether the assistance we provided actually went to those counties the Chinese had chosen.

As the negotiations continued, I saw how the Chinese viewed the negotiated document more as a starting point rather than an agreement by which they were bound. The ICPD PoA typified this approach. First, my counterparts staked out their national position, and then declared how this was in accord with the PoA.[71] It was not the reverse whereby the starting point was the international agreement and what your government then needed to do in order to honour it. In common with many sovereign states, the Chinese interpreted global conventions in a way that best suited their national interests. So it was that Peng Peiyun could call on the global community to recognise the steps the Chinese had made in reducing their population growth. By declaring China's adherence to the ICPD PoA, she could ignore the basic contradiction between individual rights and a state-administered FP programme. Was this in keeping with the Taoist Chinese philosopher Laozi in following the "way"?[72] Perhaps it was more akin to the Confucian dictum that people can be made to follow rather than made to understand.[73]

Language was always an issue whether it arose from a genuine misunderstanding or was used manipulatively. Even if English was spoken by both sides, the Chinese would speak in Chinese and we would speak in English. Translation would then take place with each translator whispering in the ear of their spokesperson. The good thing about translation is that it gave me time to think. To be avoided, however, was turning and speaking directly to your translator and not the highest-ranking official sitting opposite to you across the coffee table. Additionally, as we went through the document, line by line, paragraph by paragraph, I came to realise the Chinese did not always understand my Australian accent. I had to be disciplined, speak slowly and clearly. Any attempt at humour was lost in translation. As others had learnt,

---

[70]'China and UNFPA: 30 years of Cooperation on Population and Development'.

[71]A not uncommon starting point for many countries when subject to international scrutiny.

[72]Gia-Fu Feng, Jane English (Translators), DOADEJING', 1980, Wildwood House, London.

[73]Edward Slingerland, CONFUCIUS ANALECTS Hackett Publishing, Indianapolis 2003, p. 81.

a giggle could mean multiple things: happy, sad, angry, embarrassed, puzzled, uneasy, shy, grieving etc. Experience helped me to figure this out.

My local UN colleagues were vital in helping me navigate Chinese mannerisms as well as providing me with insights into how the thinking of my counterparts was progressing. But because the local staff were appointees from key ministries, I knew they were required to report back to their government colleagues. However, despite the obvious conflicts of interest, I never doubted that they were honest brokers. This did not mean they were not conflicted between their loyalty to UNFPA, its principles and government policy. I certainly needed to be mindful of the pressures on the staff when working within an authoritarian environment on sensitive matters such as human rights.

In 1997, after two years of negotiations, the wording in the document was beginning to take shape. The process was long and hard meaning our ongoing programme stalled pending finalisation of a new agreement.[74] But activities did continue with Chinese support but no UNFPA funding. In part, this was inevitable given that the ICPD POA, with its emphasis on individual rights, was a major departure from the previous statist approaches.[75] During a visit to Beijing from our Asia and Pacific Division Director, he explained to our Chinese counterparts four major shifts in the underlying principles.[76] First, women's health was now the driving force for FP, not the reliance on demographic goals and contraceptive methods. Second, there was recognition "…of the basic right of all couples and individuals to decide freely and responsibly the number, spacing and timing of their children and to have the information and means to do so…free of discrimination, coercion and violence."[77] Third, the UN system would benefit from greater involvement of NGOs with their skills and resources being used more efficiently in the field. Fourth, there was to be more vetting of international covenants at country level by the Executive Board. For all these reasons, UNFPA's presence in China had to be justified.

In light of this we again made it clear that UNFPA was not going to selectively apply the new ICPD principles just to accommodate the Chinese. Dr.

---

[74]Friends of UNFPA "*The Process of U.S. Funding to UNFPA*", p. 1.

[75]In retrospect the change was one more of language rather than substance. Notwithstanding that the Chinese understanding of human rights is more of a collective concept as distinct from an individualistic favoured in the West. See Chap. 9 in this book, p. XX.

[76]Notebook 6, p. 12.

[77]"The Politics of Population: Cairo 1994", p. 126.

Sadik was very aware of international women's groups and concerned governments who trusted that UNFPA would apply the POA. Although she was a friend to China, she needed to be convinced that any agreement reached would not violate ICPD. Dr. Sadik knew she would have a difficult time with the Executive Board and, as a consequence, had to be sure of China's support in order to defend our programme. My mission was to find a way that allowed her to say our support to China was genuinely in support of ICPD.[78] Our goal was to see how we could help China try out these new international approaches in selected counties which, if successful, could be used in other areas. Finally it was agreed. Twenty poor counties were proposed with a population of 8–10 million people. Coordination was to be the responsibility of DIR and MOFTEC with implementation by SFPC, in collaboration with the MOH. If successful, we would expand.

This shift in approach to FP was radically different from China's previous methods. But that wasn't the end of the story. Further complicating matters was that decisions to change policies was not within the authority of any single ministry. There were many players involved. To try and explain the ICPD approach to them all I introduced an annual planner for placement on the office walls of each of our partners throughout the country. Around the edges I had quotes from "Quality of Care" advocates and human rights activists written in Chinese. The aim was to familiarise our project personnel with a broader definition of what they were doing and make commonplace standards, regarded as normal elsewhere throughout the world, goals for them to attain.

Nonetheless, despite these initiatives and the support of a number of key Chinese demographers, the government was adamant that our final document would contain no references to "changing" or UNFPA "funding a shift". It was all about "strengthening" and "supporting their approach". Because consensus needed to come from a number of different government bodies the ultimate decision would be at the discretion of the top echelons of the Communist Party. Such a process prompted Dr. Sadik to insist that the final document be "squeaky clean" and free of any loopholes.[79]

These respective positions meant more months of negotiation as we went back and forth over wording. It wasn't always a struggle for power where UNFPA and the government were positioned in opposition to each other. But questions did arise over who had the ultimate authority to amend provincial regulations and the links between these and county implementation. There

---

[78]Notebook 6, p. 12.
[79]Notebook 7, p. 9–10.

were also matters of trust around commitments given and fears from HQ's that the Fund was being duped by Chinese undertakings given but never intended to be honoured. "No", insisted the SFPC representatives, "whatever is promised will be applied".

Strengthening our position was the fact that we were a UN organisation not a bilateral agency with national interests. We never saw ourselves in this vein, nor did the Chinese. Ours was the joint occupancy of a co-dependent space where, despite our differences and divergences, we could dialogue. Was this good relations or as the Chinese say "*Guanxi*"?[80] Yes, it was. The outcome was important to both parties.

Despite the oft-repeated reference to being "old friends", which was true and would always hold us in good stead, there seemed to be a limit to this amity. At times this could take the form of a snarled insistence about what had to be but this was an exception. However, there was an opaque barrier that was never crossed. Unlike Ghana where we often were invited to people's homes, to socialise and drink together with our counterparts, my Chinese contacts were restricted to the office or a private room in a restaurant. While these meetings were pleasant they underlined the fact that individual friendships with foreigners were off-limits.

For someone negotiating with government, the bureaucratic structure was something one could not ignore. China is, after all, a highly structured society where the political bureau of the communist party still holds the ultimate power. Today, many commentators refer to it as a "Market/Leninist" state with very aggressive party-backed capitalists, instead of a purely "Marxist/Leninist" one. This conundrum was personalised for me in a joke I was told in Beijing concerning Bush snr, Gorbachev, and Deng, who, when driving together, came to a T-intersection and argued about which way to turn. Bush snr declared, "We must turn right". "*Nyet*" said Gorbachev "We must turn left". Deng, aiming to compromise, declared, "*Bu Xing*"[81], we will indicate right, then, when safe to do so, we will turn left!". This personified the government's approach to family planning. Publicly, when it came to social engineering the central government saw population control as pivotal to ensuring economic progress and, thereby, their continued legitimacy. Privately, they were prepared to implement new ways of doing things.

---

[80] "*Guanxi*", a concept which correlates well to the English phrase "it's not what you know, it's who you know". However, as practised in China it carries more weight. Thus, toasting together and acclamations of friendship are manifestations of wanting to strengthen relations.

[81] "*Bu Xing*" (不行) literally meaning, "not o.k."

After all the back and forths the wording of our new country programme came together, and we thought, if all went well, we could begin in 1998. If not, the gap between programmes would be too long.[82] The most important element now was the so-named *32 County Programme* (increased from 20) in 22 provinces with a population close to 20 million. Whilst careful not to call it a "model" project, the Chinese rejecting the notion that an international organisation would be setting policy for a national initiative, the Government was prepared to "grope for stones to cross the river" (Deng Xiaoping's famous maxim). Being pragmatic, if it worked, they would use it. If it didn't, it would be thrown out. I was not unhappy. As argued for in my earlier assignments, when it came to changing government policy and people's sexual and reproductive behaviour, fewer initiatives were better than many because major political and cultural transitions always took time.

In the counties chosen the Chinese agreed to lift acceptor targets. The concerned provinces, while still pursuing overall demographic targets, also agreed to lift birth quotas. As a result, a couple could now have their authorised one, two or three children, whenever they liked. But, if you had more, 'social costs' would still be levied. The project also sought to establish a client-oriented reproductive health approach that would provide a wider range of quality health services, encompassing maternal health care, treatment for reproductive tract infections and sexually transmitted diseases (STDs), and a broad range of contraceptive methods not just IUDs and sterilisations.

In January 1998, the UNFPA Executive Board approved a *Fourth Programme of Assistance (1997–2000)* for the People's Republic of China.[83] One year later, in an address given in the Netherlands, Hillary Clinton stated how pleased she was "…that UNFPA and the Chinese government have recently developed a pilot program in 32 counties to address concerns (that too many women were forced to have sterilizations and abortions), to promote voluntary family planning and seek to remove all coercive actions by local officials."[84] I suspect the Chinese were even more pleased. Our approach

---

[82]Notebook 7, p. 1.

[83]The success of the programme was beyond expectations. There was a downward trend in the abortion ratio, a shift in the method mix from permanent to temporary methods, and a positive change in the levels of individual RH/FP knowledge and attitudes especially among young people. The shift from an administrative FP approach to an integrated, client-oriented approach emphasizing quality of care was said to be so pronounced that the US State Department's 2004 Human Rights Report noted that "800 other counties also removed the target and quota system and tried to replicate the UNFPA supported-product model by emphasizing quality of care and informed choice of birth control methods," potentially reaching 400 million people across China…"

[84]Address by Hillary Rodham Clinton to the Cairo Plus Five Forum, Netherlands Congress Centre, The Hague, The Netherlands, February 9, 1999.

was vindicated. My job was done. It was time to move on. Headquarters beckoned.

My story is neither an exhaustive nor scholarly history of the China FP programme nor of the UNFPA debate surrounding it. It is an uneven narrative of my five years of being stationed in Beijing and travelling throughout the country. Although, following my departure from Beijing, I was never asked at headquarters for advice or to comment on the China programme, I continued to monitor the evolution of their FP policy. Indeed, since those years I have learnt a great deal more about its history. Given the importance of the topic and the controversy surrounding it, there is much more documentation currently available than during my time. Even the regulations which were once closely guarded by the provincial authorities are now translated into English and widely available. Moreover, the controversy surrounding the FP programme has greatly diminished. There is even a muted appreciation for what the Chinese have achieved in reducing population numbers, despite its affront to human rights—something of a double standard which flies in the face of international universalism. Today, following the amended provincial regulations of 2016 allowing couples to have two children,[85] (and now three as at June 2021) I anticipate that the controversy surrounding the programme will be reduced even further. Given three decades of persuasion and propaganda leading to a national mind-set of acceptance plus a family planning bureaucracy whose vested interest is resistant to any significant change,[86] it is still hard to see the government completely abandoning its policy. Indeed, the policy has now become law, a "fundamental state policy" enshrined in the constitution.[87]/[88] Nonetheless, there remain enormous population challenges to be faced fraught with many ethical and practical dilemmas.

---

[85]It was at the 18th Central Committee of the Chinese Communist Party, October 2015, that the decision was made to abolish the one-child policy. Subsequently, following the provincial revisions made in 2016, the average TFR estimated by the UN Population Division for the period 2016–2018 was 1.6, significantly below the level of replacement. For a quarter of a century, China's fertility decline has closely resembled that of South Korea, Taiwan, Thailand, Singapore, and Viet Nam. In common with those countries, it is unlikely that the hoped-for fertility surge to counter an aging population and a declining workforce, will eventuate. Just as elsewhere couples are marrying later, delaying the age for first birth, and considering the costs of having children. Rapid urbanisation, as a result of rural migration, also impacts adversely on fertility.

[86]"If we don't achieve the family planning targets, we will have our salaries cut, face administrative punishments and have little hope of future promotion" Wang told USA Today... authorities across China collect more than US$3 billion a year from "out-of-policy" pregnancies, according to the China Economic Weekly Magazine, Calum MacLeod, op cit.

[87]In September 2018 China abolished all three family planning-related departments and created a new department titled the "Department of Demographic surveillance and Family Development" (Li Ruohan, Global Times, 2018/9/11). The emphasis now is to encourage young Han couples to have more babies although concern still remains about undeveloped areas and poverty alleviation.

[88]Yanzhong Huang op cit.

Among those dilemmas are first and foremost the imbalance of sex ratios at birth which in 2010 was an unnatural 118.4 males per 100 females,[89] and which in 2013 had only slightly changed at 115.7.[90] This imbalance of the sexes has led to the prevalence of infanticide, selective abortion, and female abandonment. Not to forget the fact that there are over 30 million fewer women in China today than would be the case if its gender balance resembled that of other countries.

The second issue is of the 'little emperors' whereby some claim that the children born under this policy are less trusting, less conscientious, less likely to take risks, less competitive, slightly more neurotic and significantly more pessimistic than before.[91] These issues are strained further by the failure of existing services to meet the needs of young people and families, as reportedly 61 million children are left behind so that their parents can work.[92]

Third, there is an obvious increase in the sex trade, possibly compounded by the millions of unmarried young men who face the prospect of not finding a wife.[93] Associated here are the increasing levels of HIV and STD infections among young people.[94]

Lastly, to absorb the 10 million new entrants to the labour market each year, China's economy needs to grow by at least 7.2%.[95] At the same time they need to maintain the balance between population, resources and the environment. Compounding this challenge is that there are now more than 230 million people aged 60 and over meaning that the 30 per cent of the

---

[89] Reference the sixth Chinese census, 2010. The global SRB average is about 105. The gap between 118 and 105 is made up of "missing girls." Explanations for this are sex-selective abortion, infanticide, delayed or late registration and non-reporting. UNFPA, 'Sex Imbalances at Birth: Current Trends, consequences and policy implications', 2012.

[90] The National Bureau of Statistics of China, '*China's Economy Showed Good Momentum of Steady Growth in the Year of 2013*', Accessed 30 November 2017, http://www.stats.gov.cn/enGLISH/PressR elease/201401/t20140120_502079.html.

[91] Rebecca Morelle "*China's one-child policy impact analysed*", BBC News, 10 January 2013.

[92] Ting Guo, '*One-in-five children are 'left-behind' by China's migrant parents*', August 20 2014, http://chinaoutlook.com/one-in-five-children-are-left-behind-by-chinas-migrant-parents/.

[93] 13.3% of the population is over 60 according to the census conducted in 2010, compared with 10.3% in 2000. Meanwhile, people under the age of 14—the country's future workers—made up 16.6% of China's population, compared with 23% a decade earlier. "Think tank calls China to adjust the one-child policy", Josh Chin, the Wall Street Journal, July 3, 2012.
"The old-age dependency ratio (the number of people above the age of 65 for every person of working age) is expected to double over the next two decades, reaching the level of Norway or the Netherlands by 2030, http://www.stats.gov.cn/enGLISH/PressRelease/201401/t20140120_502 079.html.

[94] "The working-age population—defined as those from 15 to 59—fell by 2.44 million to 920 million and is expected to fall through to 2030. The first decline in almost 50 years", The Economist, March 16, 2013.

[95] Ross Gittins, "*How China's fortunes are changing*", Sydney Morning Herald, August 2, 2014.

population in paid work will increasingly bear the tax burden.[96] How the Chinese navigate their way through these population challenges remains one of the great developmental undertakings of our age.

---

[96]The National Bureau of Statistics of China, 'Statistical Communiqué of the People's Republic of China on the 2016 National Economic and Social Development', February 28 2017, Accessed 6 December 2017, http://www.stats.gov.cn/english/PressRelease/201702/t20170228_1467503.html.

8

Surviving in the People's Paradise: DPRK

In 2021, UNFPA celebrated 36 years of cooperation with North Korea

The state-owned airline, Koryo Air, was one of only two carriers operating between Beijing and Pyongyang in the 1990s. In 1993 I was on board a Koryo flight leading a delegation of UNFPA colleagues to the Democratic People's Republic of Korea (commonly known as North Korea, hereafter DPRK). On boarding, the flight attendants directed us to sit in 'business class'. It may have been only a two-hour flight but we were pleased to receive this 'upgrade'. Unfortunately, however, we were not to enjoy the privilege for long. No sooner had we stowed our bags and sat down, we were told to relocate. Military officials were boarding the plane and due to their 'esteem', we were asked to join the other passengers in the seating allocated to workers—economy class. So began my first lesson in DPRK politics. The military came first. The tone was set for my multiple visits to the hermit kingdom.

During the flight, I browsed through the inflight magazine, which was dedicated exclusively to the exploits of the Great Leader, Kim Il Sung. The cult of personality was clearly alive, even before we had arrived. This was reinforced when a stewardess asked if we knew anything about the Great Leader or if we wanted any educational material about him. When one colleague replied that he would like to know more, the stewardess sat with him and delivered a sermon of which any evangelist would be proud. As she spoke I noticed that most of the other passengers were carrying bouquets of flowers.

© The Author(s), under exclusive license to Springer Nature
Switzerland AG 2021
I. Howie, *Reflections on a United Nations' Career*, Springer Biographies,
https://doi.org/10.1007/978-3-030-77063-1_8

How nice, I thought, they are bringing them home to present to their waiting relatives.

Upon arriving at Pyongyang airport, we were met by our host organisation, our North Korean staff,[1] and officials from other ministries. There were also a number of Mercedes vehicles waiting to ferry us into the city. To our surprise, we found the interiors of these had been stripped down, with carpet replaced by linoleum and most of the internal features missing. Was this a security measure? As we drove into the city, everything was in complete darkness. Our hosts explained that this was a security measure because the Korean War had only ended with an armistice and could re-ignite with an American attack at any time. We drove on, eventually alighting at a car park atop, what I later knew was Mansu Hill. In the lengthening shadows we could see other cars, as well as recognise other passengers from our flight. We followed our hosts, and along with the growing crowd walked out to behold an enormous bronze statue of Kim Il Sung, hand on hip and arm outstretched. We then lined up, and one by one, all the passengers approached the statue, bowed their head, and placed those boquets of flowers at its foot. That's what they were for, those bunches on the plane. But we had none. Quickly, my host gave me a bouquet, so I followed the others, approached the statue and joined the procession. Over the next five years I would repeat this ritual at the start of all my visits to Pyongyang. Like it or not, it was a key part of the elaborate, entrenched practice of paying homage to the leader and showing the utmost respect for the system.

Later, at the hotel, it was no different. Large, full-body portraits of the Great and Dear Leaders hung in the foyer. Smaller representations were in each room. The rooms were traditional and plain, linoleum floors with a large bed, a thin mattress, folded quilt and a long sausage pillow. Hot water was supplied in a thermos with loose leaf tea It came with small, floral cups and sauces. Overhead hung one fluorescent light. There was a television that had, as I discovered, three black and white channels all depicting chapters from the life of the Great Leader. There was a news channel, a channel dramatising one of the Great Leader's victories against the Japanese occupiers, and a channel broadcasting the Great Leader's visit to an agricultural cooperative. On that first night, tired from the journey, I went to bed intrigued by what new phenomena I would encounter in the coming days.

---

[1] During my time, one UNDP staff member was charged with handling the UNFPA portfolio for which we paid a proportion of his salary. Later, national staff were seconded from the Ministry of Foreign Affairs for the position of National Programme Officer, the Finance and Administration Associate and Secretarial roles. The driver was seconded from the General Bureau for Affairs with Diplomatic Missions.

Next morning I woke to the sound of singing soaring through my window. The public loudspeaker was broadcasting martial music so uniformed children could march to school singing songs of praise to the Great Leader. This was a cult of personality at its most extreme. It gave me pause to ask: what did I know about the 'People's Paradise'?

The Korean Peninsula is geographically closest to China, Russia, and Japan, all of which have impacted on Korea's history. Traditionally, Korea existed as a single sovereign political entity but Chinese cultural influences are evident in early Korean agrarian society. These are said to date from the late seventh century. In its attempts to consolidate itself as a regional power, Japan saw Korean independence as a buffer against China. Japan ousted China from Korea in the 1890s. Upon the Russian invasion of Korea in 1904, Japan declared war on Russia, vowing to 'defend and preserve the integrity and independence of Korea'.[2] Following the defeat of the Russians, the subsequent agreement of 1905, signed in and overseen by the US, assigned the management of Korean foreign affairs to the Japanese government. A Resident General was sent to Seoul but when Korean officials rejected his propositions, a significant increase of the Resident General's power placed Korea under the protectorate of Japan. This led to inevitable annexation in 1910. Oppressive Japanese imperialism was to follow.

With the 1919/20 Paris Peace Conference, at the end of WWI, the Korean people had a chance to plead their plight. However, Japanese occupiers prevented officials from obtaining passports to travel to Paris. Instead, a delegation of Koreans who had escaped Japanese rule, often farmers who had emigrated to China and Eastern Siberia, presented the newly formed League of Nations with a case for liberating Korea from Japan and restoring its independent status. Some condemned Japan and the inaction of the US saying, 'Japan agreed to…defend the independence of Korea. But see what happened a scant six years later!… [the treaty] was thrown into the wastepaper basket by the men of Tokyo, nothing came from Washington, not even a word of remonstrance'.[3] The delegates, sitting in Europe, far removed from Korea and not knowing the facts of the situation there, did not pursue the issue stating '[the] Korean problem did not come within the purview of the conference'.[4] Korea would not enter the League of Nation's radar again until the Japanese invasion of Manchuria. Korea would not be free of Japanese supremacy until its surrender at the end of World War II.

---

[2]Bonsal, S 2001, SUITORS AND SUPPLIANTS: THE LITTLE NATIONS AT VERSAILLES, Simon Publications, Safety Harbour, p. 268.

[3]Ibid., p. 268.

[4]Ibid., P. 269.

Korea was an agrarian society, but Japanese imperialism saw shifts to industrialisation and mobilisation of the military to assist Japanese war efforts. Rapid urbanisation also characterised the period, so not only was there a 'profound transformation of the Korean economy at the time'[5] but also social adjustments as most no longer lived in the province they were from. 'Colonial bureaucracy was indeed a powerful instrument of social change, coercion and extraction that was turned to imperial ends'[6] which is why people have considered the development that took place in the period "abortive [and] fractured."[7]

With the Japanese surrender in 1945 came an 'abrupt end' to their empire in China, Southeast Asia and the Korean peninsula.[8] The Allies agreed ending Japanese control was essential and a four-power trusteeship over Korea was decided upon at the Yalta Conference in early 1945. Any American hope for unilateral occupation of Korea was destroyed when Russia joined the allies to fight Japan. Further negotiations at the conclusion of World War II at the Potsdam Conference, July-August 1945, reached no definitive arrangements on Korea's future, and Korea 'loomed large as a potential trouble spot in the far-east'.[9] It was not until the Americans proposed a plan for temporary partition choosing the 38th parallel as the line of division with two occupation zones, drafted by Colonels Dean Rusk and CH Boesteel and accepted by Stalin, that some progress was made. At a later Foreign Ministers' Conference the partition plan along with procedures for Korean independence became 'General Order Number One'. A representative cross-section of Korean leaders would be selected to form a provisional government under a joint Soviet-American commission until elections could be held.

Over the following two years, each power pursued policy unilaterally, in order to mould a government in Korea favourable to their interests. When negotiation yielded no results, the matter was brought before the UN General Assembly. The US proposed an international commission to supervise elections for a provisional government. This was adopted; however, the Soviets

---

[5]Haggard S, Kang, D and Moon, CI 1997, "*Japanese Colonialism and Korean Development: A Critique*", *World Development*, vol. 25, no. 6, p. 867.

[6]Ibid., p. 868.

[7]Cummings, B 1990, THE ORIGINS OF THE KOREAN WAR, Princeton University Press, Princeton, p. 16, 54, 67.

[8]Reynolds, D 2000, ONE WORLD DIVISIBLE: A GLOBAL HISTORY SINCE 1945, Penguin Books, London, p. 38.

[9]McCune, GM 1947, "Post-war government and politics of Korea", *The Journal of Politics,* vol. 9, no. 4, p. 605.

failed to cooperate, leaving Korea 'slated for indefinite occupation.'[10] In the South, whilst the political-left enjoyed a strong popular following, this was suppressed by a US-sponsored, politically-right, military government, which had more power due to its wealth and political control. Meanwhile in the North Stalin fostered soviet-style structures and the creation of a provisional People's Committee. The appointed chairman was Kim Il Sung, known as a renowned communist guerrilla fighter during the Japanese occupation, who had spent time in the Soviet Union. He later become premier of the soon to be formed Democratic People's Republic of Korea and declared its supreme ruler. The idea of unified independence was abandoned. Amid the emerging Cold War animosity, political and security concerns were prioritised. This resulted in the creation of two separate states, the Republic of Korea (hereafter South Korea) and the DPRK. The two countries then embarked on remarkably different patterns of development. A fortified frontier was established which exists to this day.

The DPRK became a one-party state led by Kim Il Sung, a pseudo-religious, political system formed based on a 'complex blend of nationalism and communism'.[11] It was underpinned by a *Suryong* (absolute or supreme leader) –centric belief system. The totalitarian Kim regime 'merge[d] religion and politics into a uniquely powerful brew'.[12] Two of the most important characteristics of the system were the reverence for the leader and the ideology of '*Juche*' or self-reliance. The principle of '*Juche*' has been described as a manifestation of xenophobic national solipsism: meaning within the DPRK the outside world did not exist. Significant too in giving the family the right to rule was the tracing of their ancestry.[13] They claimed lineage to the sacred and still active volcano Mount Paektu located in the far north of the country. Encapsulating the ideology were the 'Ten Principles for the Establishment of the One-Ideology System' mandating unwavering support for Kim Il Sung. Not only do the people have to abide by these actions daily, evaluation meetings are held, every two days and two weeks, where everyone must report on their adherence to the principles.

In the immediate period after the partition, economic and population growth rates were lower in the DPRK than in South Korea. The population of the North was roughly half the size of the South. Its government prioritised

---

[10]Ibid., p. 609.

[11]Reynolds, *One world Divisible*, p. 38.

[12]Macintyre, B 2010, 'Young Kim Jong-un to complete Unholy Trinity', *The Australian*, http://www.theaustralian.com.au/news/world/young-kim-jong-un-to-complete-unholy-trinity/news-story/61b3aae196e42467c564969646d04e53, viewed 20 April 2016.

[13]Lee J H 2017, 'Inside Kim Jong-un's Bloody Scramble to Kill Off His Family', *Esquire Magazine*, http://www.esquire.com/news-politics/a56628/kings-of-communism/, viewed 03 Sep 2017.

the advancement of heavy industry. A 'state controlled socialist economy'[14] was implemented with the Soviets becoming the critical trade partner and supporter of the economy. However, Soviet exploitation of resources hindered the DPRK's development. There were also much slower rates of urbanisation than in the South, and by the mid-1990s thirty per cent of DPRK citizens were still rural.

In June 1950, when Kim Il Sung attacked South Korea and the war began, any further development was prevented from taking place. Initially, the DPRK had overwhelming success, soon controlling all but the south-east corner of the peninsula. This particularly alarmed the Americans who brought the matter to the UN Security Council. At the time, the Soviet Union was boycotting the UN due to issues surrounding China and so a series of resolutions were successfully passed. The first acknowledged the attack by the North Koreans and demanded a retreat by them back to the 38th parallel. When this was ignored, further resolutions necessitated help for South Korea in repelling the attack. A unified command consisting of a 15-nation coalition was formed. Under the appointed US General MacArthur, it successfully pushed the DPRK troops back to the 38th parallel. The US saw this as a unique opportunity to diminish DPRK power and continued fighting beyond the parallel almost to the border of China. At this point, the US hoped reunification under the regime of the south would be possible but instead the Chinese supported a counterattack. A stalemate then ensured. With the original border in place, an armistice in July 1953 saw an end to the fighting. However, in the absence of a peace treaty, the conflict was still officially ongoing.[15] This reality continued to shape the behaviour of both the DPRK and South Korea, informing policy and conduct; just like we saw, or rather didn't see, as we drove through the darkened city of Pyongyang in 1993.

What was UNFPA's connection with this country? We had been active there since 1985, eight years before my first visit. My preparatory reading indicated that DPRK had had an unusual pattern of population development. The war caused great cost to human life, particularly for the North, which had a smaller population and suffered higher casualties than the South. Population growth stalled as fertility rates decreased and mortality rates increased. However, population recovery, which is common in post-war booms, saw dramatic increases from 1955 to 1970 following improved

---

[14] Kim, D 1994, 'The demographic transition in the Korean peninsula, 1910–1990: South and North Korea compared', *Korean Journal of Population and Development*, vol. 23, no. 2, p. 131.
[15] Walsh, B 2009, *GCSE Modern History*, 3rd ed., Hodder Education, London.

health care and a spike in fertility rates as high as 6.4 births per woman.[16] A steady decline then started but this was reversed in the late 1980s when those born during the period of peak increase reached child-bearing age. Today, the population still has not reached 'stabilisation'[17] due to the constant turmoil in living conditions. The UNFPA's first initiative saw resources allocated to the nation's first ever population census conducted in 1989. The UNFPA found that the DPRK hospital and clinic network was well developed, including services for maternal care. However, because reproductive health and contraception were unfamiliar,[18] the Fund initiated projects in these areas as well as broader women's issues. For example, on my first visit we discussed how issues of gender equality could be introduced into the curriculum of Kim Il Sung University. Seminars and workshops were held but significant economic decline and natural catastrophes saw our efforts redirected although reproductive health continued to be emphasised.

The collapse of Moscow-dominated communism in the early 1990s, following the fall of the Berlin Wall in 1989, had a huge impact on the DPRK's economy. The Soviet Union was a major trading partner and provider of agricultural and other subsidies. Imports from the Soviet Union plummeted from $1.97 billion to just $580 million by 1991.[19] The DPRK was unable or unwilling to purchase grain in international markets. Due to animosity towards communist states, the United States had also imposed an embargo which restricted trade options. A lack of market incentives further hampered economic growth. This decline would be the precursor to an economic crisis and famine defined by the 'three shortages': that of foreign exchange, energy and food.

When I arrived in 1993, starvation was already widespread. It was estimated that only 16% of households had enough food. Although the severity of the crisis was not acknowledged by the government, and Pyongyang had largely been spared, its impact was inadvertently revealed to me. One day I was walking in the park at the back of my hotel and was puzzled by the sight of people cutting the lawns with scissors. "You would think they could use a motor mower," I said to my Chinese colleagues, "or even a hand mower". They reflected for a moment. Then it came back to them. Yes, they knew why

---

[16]Kim, DS 1994, "The demographic transition on the Korean Peninsula 1910–1990: South and North Korea compared", *Korea Journal of Population and Development*, vol. 23, no. 2, pp. 131–155.

[17]That is, a steady rate of population growth necessary to maintain a good quality of life.

[18]Lee, H, Ahn, DY, Choi, Soyoung et al. 2013, "The role of major donors in health aid to the Democratic People's Republic of Korea", *Journal of Preventative Medicine and Public Health*, vol. 46, no. 3, pp. 118–126.

[19]Lee, D 2006, THE NORTH KOREAN FAMINE AND FOOD SHORTAGE: THE PROBLEM, THE POLITICS AND THE POLICY, Harvard Law School, Harvard.

the citizens were cutting the grass. Their parents had told them that during Mao's 'Great Leap Forward' in the 1950s when people were hungry, the urban dwellers had resorted to keeping rabbits in their apartments. They were a source of protein and grew rapidly. They then discovered that to keep them fed there was nothing better than the fresh green grass shoots so abundant in the public parks. What we were seeing now, was a repetition of an old survival mechanism. The North Koreans were keeping rabbits in their apartments. I was shocked, particularly as this was Pyongyang, the privileged capital where only fifteen per cent of the population lived. These were the elites classified with a high 'songbun' (a societal ranking system based on family background and political standing). Starvation had to be worse in rural areas. It was as I soon discovered.

Throughout this period notes from my visits to the countryside consistently described the food situation as 'at crisis proportions', 'only getting worse', 'deteriorating' and becoming 'country-wide'. Coping mechanisms I heard about included eating wild roots, even though many people became violently ill or died, scavenging through garbage and engaging in illicit black-market trade. However, just as the people of Pyongyang were resourceful in finding solutions to their lack of food so too were the rural population. Another UN colleague whose assignment saw him travel in the disadvantaged northern provinces, told me how clandestine enterprises such as pop-up restaurants serving dog-meat stew, were an emerging sight. That said, he still recalled seeing many orphans whose parents were so weak from the lack of food that they had died from TB and other respiratory diseases. These children would roam in gangs begging, often targeting tourist buses from China. The train stations were a hub for them, he said, where they scavenged among the crowds travelling to their relatives or other towns or the border, in a desperate search for food or a means to defect.

Natural disasters compounded the situation when crop land and infrastructure were destroyed and the unavailability of seed affected agricultural recovery. However, the principal impediment to improving the food situation was the Kim regime and its policy and priorities. According to my colleagues from the World Food Programme the government directly discriminated against parts of the population, prevented necessary reform, and rendered the efforts of the UN and other humanitarian donors less effective. It continually cut public rations upon which much of the population depended. Farmers who were usually self-sufficient had their reserves taken from them for storage in collective warehouses. While shortages were evident in the early 1990s it was not until 1994 that Kim Il Sung publicly admitted that people were hungry. He announced a 'two meals a day' campaign, calling on citizens to cut out a daily meal. Internally, the famine was referred to as the 'Arduous March'. Despite the evident failure of the agricultural system there was no decision to make reform and introduce policy to alter production or distribution. The regime's steadfast dedication to its own systems prevented alternative approaches to tackling the severe food shortages. Kim Il Sung was recorded saying to Deng Xiaoping 'if you open the window the flies will come in...if we let them in then the economy will get out of control. We will lose control'.[20] The *Juche* principle, which underpinned society, meant the DPRK was closed to any foreign ways of doing things. It was not until 1998 that UNFPA managed to assign a Chinese consultant to the agricultural sector.

The government's expenditure priorities not only neglected the food shortages, but also energy and economic crises. Following natural disasters in the far north, power stations received limited supply. My UN colleague remembers having to be ready with candles as blackouts were everywhere and could be expected at any time. There was no transport and bicycles, previously banned, were brought from the Chinese border. The signs of economic hardship in Pyongyang were the most telling as it was the showpiece of the 'People's Paradise'. Indicators I saw included large department stores attended by bored sales assistants and mostly empty shelves as even the wealthier citizens could not afford the products. The large hotel construction, pyramidal in shape, which dominated the Pyongyang skyline, was an empty shell and, with no resources to complete the building's interior,[21] was abandoned with one solitary guard at its entrance.

Households were mandated one 45-watt bulb for each room and, to ensure compliance, curtains were required to remain open at all times. Privacy was not an option. As you walked at night you wondered who these dimly lit figures were as they flitted across the windows. Streetlights were also off, ostensibly as a precaution against US air attacks although this may have had more to do with an absence of power. There were few trams and those that were running were overcrowded. In their absence, walkers shuffled by in the darkness, head down, valiantly stepping out the 10,000 m the Great Leader

---

[20] Kim Il Sung cited in Human Rights Council. 2014, *Report of the detailed findings of the commission of inquiry on human rights in the Democratic People's Republic of Korea*, United Nations, Geneva, p. 180.

[21] Construction of the Ryugyong Hotel began in 1987 but the economic crisis of the early 1990s was said to have prevented it from being completed, or as I was told it had more to do with a fault in the foundations or an absence of power to drive the lifts. Rumours abounded. Construction was resumed in 2008 with a plan to open in 2012. Although the exterior is complete, the hotel still remains unopened.

encouraged as daily exercise. Even I shuffled alongside them in the winter months, shrunk into my thick, down-filled ex Chinese military-coat to escape the fierce winds. It was a city of shadows.

But the absence of public amenities was not reflected in the state of military preparedness. You saw soldiers everywhere, walking among the masses, labouring in work crews, bringing in the harvest, being transported somewhere and always goose-stepping in those massive military parades. Military preparedness was vital both as defence mobilisation and as a means of reinforcing authority. I was constantly told how the DPRK must never appear weak, and be always ready for an attack. Given this siege mentality, the image of the Kim family, as powerful, unifying rulers, was critical. By extension, when Kim Il Sung died in 1994, what better way to promote the continuing strength of the regime, at a time of uncertainty, than to deify the regime's founding father? Thus, the harrowing outpouring of public grief at the death of their 'spiritual father'.

In order for the masses to pay homage to the 'Great Leader', the authorities constructed a mausoleum in which to house his body, along with a new railway line and station. Communist leaders including Stalin, Mao and Ho Chi Minh had all been embalmed and this was deemed an appropriate way to honour the eternal president. We were soon to have the honour of paying homage.

Late one night we were told to be prepared early the next morning for a very special occasion. As distinguished guests, we were invited to view Kim Il Sung's mausoleum named the 'Kumsusan Palace of the Sun', before its opening to the public.[22] We were to dress soberly in a suit and tie. At 8 o'clock the following day, the ever-reliable Mercedes were there, ferrying us through the empty streets to the edge of a vast quadrangle in which was housed the mausoleum. As we alighted, we were told to line up in a triangular formation with me at the front, two behind, three and then four. Two goose-stepping soldiers, their weapons shoulder borne, waited to lead us across the quadrangle. At the given signal, we were under way.

When we neared the building, two large heavy-set doors opened automatically. We stepped inside to be greeted by a blast of air coming down upon us, presumably to remove any contamination. Once inside, we were directed across the marble floor to another series of doors and then beyond to yet another. They all mysteriously opened as if by magic. The lighting was dimmed, solemn music played, and the atmosphere was one of reverence. We finally came to the inner sanctum in the middle of which was a

---

[22]The railway station being especially built for the purpose of transporting in the masses was not finished.

glass cabinet containing the embalmed body of Kim Il Sung. What to do next? My colleagues looked to me as did our hosts. I walked to the sarcophagus, bowed my head, paused, waited, and then repeated this action at the remaining three sides of the body. The others did exactly the same. They walked to each corner, bowed, and presumably reflected in a moment of silence. I then proceeded to walk out backwards keeping my eyes focused on the 'Great Leader'. The others did likewise, thankfully without stumbling into each other and causing a diplomatic incident.

Once outside the chamber, we turned around and proceeded to exit the building. But to our surprise, when we reached the entrance chamber, there was a television crew, arc lights on and a very large condolence book, opened at a fresh page for me to declare my thoughts. I proceeded to write. No sooner had I finished than my English words were translated into Korean and read to the adoring public, no doubt eagerly following this momentous event on television. Like it or not, we had become pawns in this vast charade of dynastic worship. The '*Suryong*' or absolute ruler and its political system was always, no matter the circumstances, the primary concern of the state. Even in death, Kim Il Sung received priority of resources. The extreme personality cult of this totalitarian regime required us to publicly pay homage, irrespective of our private views. Whilst we could see the disturbing aspects of the situation, we were equally drawn in.

That the public infrastructure was under stress was visible. Not only were the buses overcrowded but the trains were old, rickety, and very basic. People were walking enormous distances burdened with heavy loads. There were virtually no cars, only trucks jammed with workers standing in the back. Despite these privations, the regime continued to portray a glowing image. Even when driving through the countryside on a moonless night, you would suddenly come across a large floodlit billboard on which was depicted a beaming 'Great Leader', arms outstretched as he embraced adoring children, all looking up into his face and all backgrounded by a field of blossoming flowers. The underground stations were also elaborately finished with guilt-edge mosaics depicting episodes in the life of the Great Leader. Every building we ever visited, no matter where its location throughout the country, contained a large portrait of the 'Great Leader' at its entrance, and smaller depictions in each room.

The leadership may have been omnipresent and eternally wise, but there was, however, a crisis of resources. There simply was not enough food. Crops had failed destroyed by unprecedented flooding. Countless numbers of people died from illnesses associated with starvation.[23] It was only in 1995 that Kim Jong Il, who succeeded his father, reached out for international aid to assist with the food crisis. Intervention at an earlier stage probably could have prevented some of the acute malnutrition particularly experienced by children. But this would have amounted to an admission of failure.

Then, once humanitarian organisations, including the UN, began supplying food aid, the regime was still not fully cooperative. For example, my UN colleagues from the World WFP were forbidden from monitoring where the aid was being distributed and had to rely on the regime for delivery. They suspected, rightly as it turned out, it was only going to those people and areas "consider[ed] crucial for maintaining the political system, and its leadership, at the expense of those deemed to be expendable,"[24] that is, the military and the élite of Pyongyang. This reality was brought home to us at a banquet, hosted by a Minister for our delegation, at the height of the famine. He asked us not to talk about the range of dishes served on our return to Beijing.[25]

Particularly affected by these diversions of food were the northern regions, where citizens of the lowest 'songbun' tended to live. These areas were strictly off-limits to foreigners, including the UN, but we knew they received minimal government assistance and little of the international aid. Donors reacted to this interference and demanded access to consumption and storage figures but again the authorities refused to provide this information.[26] Because many donors operated under a 'no access no aid' principle, this meant people in the north were most severely affected by the famine. Other donors would not give rice knowing that it would be misused. Still more were only willing to give corn, even though children and the elderly needed a more balanced diet.[27]

The lack of appropriate behaviour and transparency made it hard for the UN and other donors to effectively implement projects. Take, for example, UNFPA's funding of the census in 1993. At the time, this accounted for over 50% of our programme resources. When the North Koreans announced they were going to conduct the census at midnight on December 31 we were surprised. We did, however, query this timing knowing that the DPRK is a

---

[23]Estimates for deaths from the famine, 1995–2000, range from 236,900 (DPRK's estimate) to 2,648,939 (highest international estimate cited in Goodkind and West 2001).

[24]Human Rights Council. 2014, *Report of the detailed findings of the commission of inquiry*, p. 172.

[25]The meal included sliced meats, vegetables, and salads.

[26]In one instance where the DPRK were caught diverting aid they claimed it was an error and re-diverted it.

[27]It is important to note that the DPRK had no previous experience handling outside supplies of foreign aid, so problems in getting food from donor through the UN system were inevitable. Neither the DPRK government nor population or workers were equipped to deal with food supplies.

mountainous country and it was the middle of winter. But who could fault their logic when they assured me the timing was optimal, as everyone was sure to be home. In preparation for the count, we provided training and technical advice. Yet, when it came to the results, they refused to reveal the findings, other than in the most general terms. The authorities continually fudged the data,[28] including the total population, so accuracy was never achieved. Much of this may have been due to security reasons. You are, after all, surrounded by enemies. It may have also been to conceal human rights abuses such as the percentage of the population in prison camps, and abductees from other countries.

The regime's resistance to transparency inhibited our access to data. We found it incredibly difficult to elicit information from the government. A worker sitting at their desk never knew what the person sitting next to them was doing, or so they said. Despite this, the same official could never travel to a UN meeting in Bangkok or elsewhere without our paying for another official to accompany him.[29] There was always a reason: translation, technical expertise, first-time travel, secretarial support. But it was widely assumed that the extra traveller was needed in order to watch the other, especially, should they want to escape.

This was made evident to us on one occasion when, on the night before my team was due to leave Pyongyang, we held a celebratory dinner in our hotel's restaurant. As we went to pay the bill, one of my colleagues discovered that her handbag was missing. Critically, the bag contained passport, two hundred American dollars and aeroplane tickets for the following day. We alerted the hotel management. Their immediate response was 'You must have left it in your room'. When none of us could find it in her room, we were then told 'She must have mislaid it. Now, you should go and rest'. We were having none of this. We advised our hosts that the handbag had been stolen and that the problem was to be solved immediately. When there were still no results by two in the morning, we determined we would not leave without our colleague and went to bed. The following morning we were thrilled to be told that the handbag had been found in the mud by the river bank. Everything was recovered except the $200 but, curiously, none of the bag's contents were wet. We did not pursue the matter any further relegating it to yet another of the unknowns of the DPRK. As such, the episode mirrored the larger reality UNFPA faced. We could never conduct our work effectively

---

[28]The DPRK is not the only country to withhold their census findings. Many other countries do for a variety of reasons.

[29]They were nearly always men.

because we lacked the necessary access, trust and flexibility. This was a senti-ment reinforced by the Swedish ambassador who said it was difficult to give advice because the government thought 'we are dangerous [and] not good for the country'.[30] In the same discussion he stated 'they never open the book for us'. He, along with the Eastern European diplomats, were our most reliable sources as their countries had long-standing relations with the DPRK, dating from the Soviet era.

This intransigence was of particular concern when it came to the challenges faced by the public health system. How could we bring best practice in light of this dogmatism? Hospitals were stretched beyond their capacities, basic medicines were lacking, and women were giving birth in very challenging circumstances. And that was only what we could observe. The authorities continued to insist that they did not need any help from us and, much like the issue of starvation, they denied having high maternal mortality, STI's and HIV/AIDS. Doing so would have pointed to failings of their leadership. However, upon learning large sums of aid money were associated with the RH cause, they altered their approach, telling us whilst AIDS <u>may</u> exist in their country, it had been introduced by foreigners. Thus, they should receive the aid earmarked to eradicate such an impure virus.

Cultural norms also prevented us from executing our programmes as we would have preferred. For example, when producing material for public dissemination regarding 'reproductive health' there was a long halt before publishing so that an appropriate term could be found. We were told that, culturally, RH was not an idea that had existed and finding the right expression, one which wouldn't offend or suggest illness, was very impor-tant. To maintain a positive working relationship with DPRK officials, we had to appease the government whilst balancing the achievement of our mandate and upholding our UNFPA values. We had to wait for decisions regarding 'political appropriateness'. Constantly facing this type of govern-ment behaviour hindered our ability to instigate programmes that were desperately needed.

We visited many maternal health clinics, at '*ri*' (rural country) or county level. What surprised us was no matter the time we were there, patients were rarely seen. Staff would conduct you around the complex, but it always felt like a staged presentation. As we had come to expect, they would explain how their procedures, routines and processes were dictated by the supreme leader on his last visit. They followed <u>his</u> direction, which was not always the most modern and effective. But, as we have seen, the *Suryong's* standing in society was so elevated, there was never any question.

---

[30]These notes were penned in my personal notebooks of the period 1995–1998.

This was true of every place we visited, whether farms, factories or centres of demography. Their approach was always informed by the instructions of one of the two leaders following their visit to the workstation. In light of this 'wisdom', any television report or image showing either one of the leaders invariably showed those surrounding them holding notebooks and pencils at the ready, waiting to write down any thoughts or instructions. There was no room for indifference or apathy. The totalitarian state required you to positively demonstrate support for the regime be it the pride you displayed by wearing the badge in your lapel on which was shown the heads of the Great and Dear Leaders or the way your children marched to school singing their praises as they were broadcast over the public address system.

In a similar vein, when the 'Great Leader' said it was good for your health to walk daily, everyone did so. This was why, we were told, so many people were walking from place to place, but the question begs whether this was true health advice or promoting certain behaviour to conceal deficiencies in public transport and development. What was evident, however, was that the supreme leader's word was taken as absolute.

The society was orientated around mass collectivism, which diminished any sense of individualism and centred everyone's behaviour on paying homage to the *Suryong*. This was deep-seated, even into the way the city was constructed. Pyongyang featured Stalinist architecture with a central square, perfect for mass gatherings, with huge portraits of historical communist figures including Stalin, Lenin, Marx and Hagel, although these would be replaced as the DPRK pursued a totally nationalistic agenda. During my visits there was and continues to be, an emphasis on public entertainment. Evidence the large parks, symbolic statues[31] and special venues where mass entertainment such as circuses and carnivals could be held. DPRK citizens also showed their dedication to the supreme leader en masse. On one occasion my wife was fortunate to experience this. She was escorted to the Grand People's Study Hall—a large building in traditional Korean style and comparable to a public library, the only difference being that your access to sections of the library was determined by your party and security pass. When my wife was shown over the building, she was taken to the rooftop in order to gain a view of the city. This happened at a time when thousands of people who we had seen earlier in the day heading towards a rallying point in front of the Study Hall, were now assembled and being directed by a man standing on a rickety fruit box, next to my wife and waving flags. She watched as he snapped the coloured flags this way and that, while the masses below

---

[31] A statue of the *Chollima*, the mythical Korean Pegasus which represents speed and perseverance, rears up over the centre of the city.

followed, creating those instant wonderful scenes. This was the positive image the North Koreans liked to project to the world. It was also a celebratory display, typifying those mass events[32] whose intention was to generate a sense of unity, geared towards the *suryong*. All this systematic propaganda enabled the DPRK to function as a monolithic state.

We also had operational barriers beyond the DPRK system when executing our programme. Not for the first time, nor the last, I became aware of the overarching mandates of the various UN agencies when it came to reproductive health. WHO and UNICEF were both operating in the DPRK but there was no coordination of plans, resources and budgets which rendered the UN's operations less efficient. Having come from Ghana I never foresaw this as an issue because there the donors and agencies agreed on a joint country plan. In the DPRK, however, I saw the challenges confronting the funds, agencies, and programmes of the UN system when it came to cohesion and cooperation. My notebooks often record frustration with the lack of coordination, resources, and information-sharing. This was a continual problem which I would eventually confront when posted to a much larger programme in Viet Nam. Another weakness was the lack of technical back-up. We had no one in-country supporting our work and coupled with the lack of communication from DPRK officials, made programme execution hard. We were not always sure when the money allotted would arrive or, if it did, would arrive on time. When it came to reports from our counterpart agency, there was none despite the efforts of the technical staff.

Additionally, the agencies did not always know how the North Korean side was bureaucratically organised. But here we had the help of our Chinese colleagues who were sympathetic to, and familiar with, the North Korean situation. Unlike many UN staff, nothing in the DPRK was a surprise to the Chinese. The organisation of state systems was very similar, and they knew what their counterparts were doing, how they made decisions and their restraints.

Despite these internal limitations, and the barriers presented by the nature of the regime, our work in the DPRK from 1993 to 1998 did improve the health and food security for many. Additionally, we trained demographers, updated their equipment and acquainted them with modern practices, invaluable for collecting data for development as well as other purposes. When I stopped visiting the country the UNFPA's work did not stop. New country programmes were constructed and more improvements in reproductive health, nutrition and food security, women's issues and demography

---

[32]For example, February 16, Kim Jong Il's birth date, is celebrated annually as the 'Day of the Shining Star'.

continued to be made. Other agencies, including the WHO and UNICEF, also continued their work and currently 6 agencies operate in the country.

In this century DPRK continues to face many of the same challenges in the domain of RH including high maternal mortality rates, weak family planning and high prevalence of RTIs. Most maternal deaths still occur in the home. In 2012 the national health survey showed the general indicators around maternal and newborn health were below target. Limitations included lack of equipment and skills at *ri* level where 43% of births take place, lack of early risk detection diagnostic skills, lack of surgical capacity at county hospitals and logistical difficulties in referral. There was also a 14.5% unmet need for family planning. Constant shortfalls in women's empowerment, HIV/AIDS and youth and adolescent sexual health were also evident but the government was unwilling to address these issues insisting they were alien.

The UNFPA Reproductive Health Care Package (2004–2006) attempted to remedy some of these challenges by training staff and providing essential drugs and equipment in 23 village clinics, 9 hospitals and 3 provincial maternal hospitals. The 2011–2014 programme was required to concentrate its efforts in South Pyongyang, Kangwon and South Hamgyong. In part, this was to deliver more effectively but was also insisted on by the government. Unfortunately, when the counties were assigned there was no means to verify whether they were areas of most need, as access was denied beyond those operation areas. New targets to reduce mortality were set for which the government's adoption of a national reproductive health strategy in 2011–2015 was important although not all aspects were adequately addressed.

In the field of demography, the principal problems continue to be a lack of trained demographers and data. A further census was completed in 2008 but the UN was still working to achieve more access to the field in order to conduct assessments and strengthen collection and analysis. Significantly, the UNFPA has never been informed what the DPRK's population policy is and, as a result, is unable to influence the policy or verify the data used.

Projects from the 2013–2016 Country Programme were geared towards achieving the Millennium Development Goals. In common with other countries they were adapted to the needs of the population, as interpreted by the government, and were in keeping with the UNFPA mandate. Reproductive health continued to be a focus. A more behavioural approach was aimed to have a long-term impact. Short-term humanitarian needs, but also long-term development strategy, were addressed. Better cooperation with the DPRK government was sought (euphemistically referred to in UN language as 'the uniting of stakeholders') and those with the highest level of need sought to be reached by UNFPA interventions.

In 2005 the DPRK was reclassified to the 'B' band, denoting it was no longer a country of priority needs. However, the economy remained fragile and DPRK continued to be susceptible to shock, with weak resilience. Energy difficulties, the weakness of infrastructure and logistical support, an imbalance in import-export policy and international sanctions contributed to the instability. As agriculture remained the backbone of the economy, this vulnerability was exacerbated. There was still high malnutrition, an underlying cause of maternal and infant mortality, despite reduced rates of stunting and wasting in pregnant and breastfeeding women. Short- and long-term interventions were made in agricultural production, nutritional support/food assistance, and prevention and treatment of malnutrition. However, critical day-to-day needs still needed to be addressed.

Despite these challenges, the government announced an end to all humanitarian programmes, but in 2011–2014 a fifth UNFPA cycle was introduced which gave rise to the current programme. The main recommendations were to continue with those areas the government supported, namely, strengthening reproductive health policy, planning and the provision of services as part of upgrading the health system. However, the UN development team continues to confront the same challenges as I did with my team: lack of transparency and access; difficulty in surmounting the dogmatic policy and procedures as laid down by the *suryong* and scrupulously followed by health workers; and cultural and linguistic barriers.

Even though the nineties were a period of great hardship, my visits were always business-like and my Korean counterparts welcoming and confident. Notwithstanding the polemics, propaganda and xenophobia, I encountered many committed people in the DPRK: doctors, nurses, statisticians, all doing their best in difficult circumstances. I was not sure, however, that this applied to our government counterparts. Witness our main government intermediary. He drove us to distraction because he simply didn't do anything. Always courteous, always promising but then nothing. When I went to complain to his superiors in the ministry I was given a fair hearing including expressions of concern for the lack of support and the need for more professional behaviour. Diplomatically I felt the message had been heard and anticipated action would be taken. I was wrong. Something was done. He was transferred to the DPRK mission to the UN in New York where some years later he gave me a cheery greeting as we met in the delegates' dining room!

Much of my recollections of the DPRK can doubtless be repeated by others who have visited the Hermit Kingdom. The difference between these and my own experience was that I had the 'neutral' status accorded to a UN official and was relatively 'free' both in my interactions with the government and my travel throughout the country. I was not treated as someone who needed to be convinced of the virtues of the DPRK regime, but rather as someone who had the best interests of the country at heart, especially of its ordinary people.

On my last visit to North Korea, I found I was struggling to maintain my diplomatic composure as I increasingly questioned the Potemkin nature of my surroundings. Still, I agreed to visit the "International Friendship Exhibition" in Hyangsan, thirty to fifty kilometres from Pyongyang. This is a museum in which all the gifts world leaders have given to Kim Il-Sung are catalogued and displayed: such is the cult of personality that the Great Leader is believed to be globally beloved. Located in a picturesque forested area at the foothills of the Myohyangsan mountain, the building was a large imposing structure softened for me, somewhat, by the autumn colours. You entered only to be immediately confronted by a large black bulletproof ZiL limousine, gifted to Kim by Joseph Stalin. Later, as we peered into the display cabinets and wandered through room after room, I asked to see any gift given by an Australian. The catalogue was opened, and pages turned as officials scanned the list. At last, a reference was found, and a guide led us down the long corridor. We climbed the stairs and then followed another corridor until we came to the right room with its assigned, glass cabinet. I peered in and there was a box of suit-pocket handkerchiefs, serrated along the top, and still in the original packaging. I looked closer at the label and recognised a large department store in my hometown of Melbourne. I asked who was the magnanimous donor. Again, the catalogue was consulted. 'Ted Hill', I was told. I vaguely knew the name and after I returned to Beijing, I enquired who Ted was. The late Ted Hill was a Melbourne barrister, and a Communist, who had fallen out with the Soviet Union, become a Maoist and pledged his support to the People's Republic as well as its close ally, the DPRK. By the size of his gift, Ted was not wholly convinced, being loath to spend too much by way of adoration, but there it was, further evidence of universal love.

By the time of my last visit, I was increasingly irritated by having to publicly endorse this cult of personality. It was time to go. Being disappointed in myself for the game I was playing, I was increasingly unable to control my frustration. I was doing the best I could, but the environment was deeply suspect. Ideologically speaking, I was becoming 'bolshie'. Engels, Hegel, Marx, Lenin, Stalin and all those founding fathers of communism hanging in the Kim Il-sung Square, may once have been of interest, but they were now gone. All that was left were the portraits of the Great Leader, the Dear Leader and now the Supreme Leader—the holy trinity. They were everywhere and everything to the North Korean people, all twenty-four million of them. They couldn't escape having to show their reverence daily, the regime all-pervasive in their lives. The country saw itself under siege, surrounded by enemies. I needed to leave this theocratic, paranoid state. It was time for others in the UN family to support the needs and aspirations of the Korean people.

9

You Must Be Mad: UN Headquarters

"When all's said and done, more will be said than done" Aesop

Day two in Manhattan, New York. It was lunchtime and I was crossing East 42nd Street about to walk down Second Avenue, a wide intersection with crowds of people moving quickly in both directions. Being new I was not sure how best to navigate the crossing. As I reached halfway, a colleague walking the opposite way leaned in towards me and declared "You must be mad!" This was not an encouraging beginning.

As with previous assignments, New York seemed not to have started well. I was already anxious prior to arrival not only because I would proceed without my wife and son who were staying on in Beijing until the end of the school year, but also because of a characteristic silence from headquarters. The Personnel Branch had neither activated the necessary visa requirements nor answered any of my emails. This only added to my apprehension about moving from the "field" to UNFPA headquarters, particularly coping with the transition from marginal scrutiny and self-reliance to one which would very likely involve "walking on eggshells",[1] now that I was directly answerable to the Executive Director.

Having spent my career in the 'field', I was unsure how I would tackle the extensive personnel manuals. I felt unprepared and not at all certain I

---

[1] As one long-term staff member described it.

© The Author(s), under exclusive license to Springer Nature
Switzerland AG 2021
I. Howie, *Reflections on a United Nations' Career*, Springer Biographies,
https://doi.org/10.1007/978-3-030-77063-1_9

© The Author(s), under exclusive license to Springer Nature
Switzerland AG 2021
I. Howie, *Reflections on a United Nations' Career*, Springer Biographies,
https://doi.org/10.1007/978-3-030-77063-1_9

could transition to this job, one where I needed to have substantive views on what was required to strengthen personnel practices. However, and somewhat altruistically, I did believe that with a well-directed plan the Office of Personnel and Training (OPT) would be better equipped to usher in a new era of empathy and commitment towards strengthening UNFPA capacity, particularly in the "field". Indeed, I hoped to become a positive voice for those I had left behind on the front line.

When I arrived at work on that first day, I found I had not been allocated an office. Surely, I thought, it was reasonable to expect some preparation for the new Chief of the OPT, even as a common courtesy. I was obliged to visit the Executive Director (ED) to ask where I should sit. Office space was then found, two floors away from my staff! But whose office was this? The incumbent eventually showed up, somewhat of a 'floater'[2] although an old hand at headquarters. He proceeded to give me a briefing, more alarming than the words expressed earlier on the pedestrian crossing. "Nobody trusts top management" he told me, "people lie to each other and to their underlings." He cited a recent survey[3] which found the majority of staff approached HR with mistrust. "The ED cannot afford anymore hiccups", my colleague warned, adding "Don't lie, be objective and make transparent decisions!"

As a final piece of advice my colleague added, "Leave the interpretation of personnel manuals to the experts in your office". This seemed a sensible option as few HR staff had ever served outside HQ and over many years had developed an encyclopaedic knowledge of operational procedures strictly according to the manual. But from a field perspective the view was that HR staff often seemed overly bureaucratic and defensive, exhibiting a kind of bunker mentality. Process driven and reactive. Because of this it soon became very clear that a key aspect of my job would require tricky negotiations between personnel interplay and politics. In fact, in my first week I was taken aside by staff members from other divisions and informed that it was 'important for me to know' there had been a great deal of negative discussion regarding OPT practices but, 'under no circumstances' could I be told who said what other than it reflected fallout from the global survey.

On the positive side, my relative unfamiliarity with HQ and its multitude of players allowed me to take a more objective stance in untangling the web

---

[2]Not attached to a fixed position in the staffing table.

[3]Biannual Global surveys of staff attitudes continue. The 2017 survey again saw DHR viewed unfavourably. Reinforced was the reality that most managers fail to fulfil their HR responsibilities and, typically, deflect them away to DHR. For most HR professionals this results in a no-win situation. They lose if they do and lose if they don't.

of distrust. The need for transformation in workplace culture quickly became a priority, a process some colleagues estimated would take the better part of a year. Meanwhile, they advised that I be content with small victories and that any changes could only be brought about through example. To this end, I began to walk the corridors, introducing myself. I announced that I was available to meet with any staff on any issue at any time. I responded in person to emails rather than replying online. I scheduled briefings with every branch. Later, at regional field meetings, I tried to meet with everyone if only for fifteen minutes each.

Some weeks later, I was still sitting in my temporary office. While the room may have been devoid of embellishment other than a desk and chair, it did have a red phone that allowed the ED to summon me immediately to her office, irrespective of what I might be doing. It rang. I startled and nervously picked up the receiver. I was summoned to the 19th floor, about to walk on those "eggshells" of which I had been warned. "I want you to appoint this young woman to a position". After taking a deep breath, I ventured to suggest this may not be a good idea especially when the potential appointee was known personally to the ED. Moreover, despite my limited knowledge in such matters and fearful of displaying my ignorance, I suggested we go through a process. "Don't we require a job description, vacancy announcement, applications, shortlisting, interviews, references and an open appointment?" "Oh", she said, "Do it your way". I believed I had successfully made my point and been given the all-clear to apply the staff appointment's process, already well-articulated in the policies and procedures manual. Then came a caveat. Follow guidelines as required but when an executive decision was requested, discuss it first in the office of the Executive Director.[4] State your case with her and when a ruling was agreed and an instruction given, publicly support the management.

To establish a *modus operandi*, I developed the practice of preparing a regular update for the ED, covering all current issues relevant to HR. We would then discuss, negotiate an agreed position and that would be the stance carried into meetings of the Executive Committee (EC) or acted upon as required.

On this procedural understanding, I attended my first meeting of the EC. Being new and keen, I arrived early and took up a position seated at the farthest end of the table from the entrance thereby allowing others to fill the

---

[4]My experience with and knowledge of other Executive Directors suggest they either follow established HR procedures when making appointments or completely override them appointing whoever they want to. This came down to the ED's perception of themselves as leader (i.e., the one who made all key decisions) plus whether or not they trusted the decisions of line managers. Depending on the practice followed, so the culture of the organisation was determined.

vacant seats. Imagine my surprise when the last person to enter before the ED came in, asked if I would swap seats so that he could sit next to her rather than in her direct line of sight. Not quite knowing why the request was made, I obliged. Later, I came to realise that in EC meetings as in many comparable power structures, there are those who want to mirror the thoughts of the leader. This is easier to do if you are sitting beside rather than opposite her.[5]

I soon came to accept that, like it or not, it was the prerogative of the ED to expect ongoing involvement in personnel matters and, on occasion, to make a unilateral political appointment. This strategy allowed her to maintain absolute control over all matters relating to staff. It was an approach that not only neutered the role of individual managers but ensured the ED was the final arbiter on personnel matters. I asked the ED if she thought this was good practice. She replied, "No, but if you give people too much warning, they will challenge your decision." The downside of this exercise of power was an apprehensive staff, obliged to curry favour and vulnerable to corridor gossip.[6]

But why did the ED want to be so involved with staff appointments and staff movements[7] as opposed to individual managers charged with HR responsibilities? I think the answer had to do with the cultural underpinning of the appointees. I was told that, in general, executive directors could not help themselves when it came to making personnel appointments, regardless of their public advocacy for procedural transparency. While this may have been the norm for a member of a privileged elite, to my mind it did not equate with modern and efficient personnel practices. Regrettably, this practice extended more broadly to appointments throughout the global UN system where they were often based on country representation, linguistic grouping (e.g., Anglophone/Francophone), regional origins and seniority, rather than merit.

Despite the existence of those lengthy personnel manuals, ambassadors and their representatives were others inclined to seek advantages for their

---

[5]Thereby mirroring the experience of staff at the League of Nations. "… It always felt good, generally speaking, to be *with* the laughter." Frank Moorhouse, COLD LIGHT, The Edith Trilogy, Vintage, Sydney, 2011, page 87.

[6]My experience mirrored even worse situations elsewhere in the system. "I was very disturbed by this stifling bureaucratic culture of WFP, with its pervasive culture of hierarchy and obsequiousness. The Executive Director was treated like a god. If he entered a meeting, even with just two or three senior colleagues, all stood, a practice which I immediately stopped. There was a reluctance to take decisions and virtually everything ended on the desk of the Executive Director…I had ended a culture of fear…" James Ingram, op cit, page 66.

[7]As of December 1997, the number of UNFPA professional staff at HQ was 98; support staff at HQ, 126; professional staff in the field, 73; support staff in the field, 390; and, national programme officers, 121. Total, 808. UNFPA staff in 2016—at HQ's 460; globally 2631; the number of country offices 139.

nationals. They would hound the ED, and me, with arguments that suggested their country representation was unaligned with their generous contributions to the Fund. Whenever a new posting was announced, I would often receive a visit from a diplomat asking why he or she had not been notified in advance. At times they would vet their nationals working for us asking why they had not been promoted or transferred. Given the regulatory impartiality of the appointment process and the need to maintain geographic balance, I tended to avoid lunches with diplomats and colleagues when it became clear they sought some favour.

At times, these ambassadors or their juniors attended meetings of the Executive Board.[8] I clearly recall my first attendance at such a meeting which always took place in the UN Secretariat Building. On that occasion our HR proposal for training was an item for debate. I had compiled information in a ring binder, colour-coded in preparation for whatever might be asked. It soon became apparent that it was mostly junior diplomats sitting behind the country flags, acting under instructions from their respective missions. Indeed, it also became apparent that the donor countries and the recipient country listed for a presentation on that day, had already made any relevant decisions in the corridors of the UN building. At this and subsequent meetings, I was often surprised at the lack of probing questions or vetting of any substance. Whatever UNFPA said was automatically accepted. I assumed, perhaps naively, that this was because of our attractive reproductive right's mandate and the strong public line taken against conservative voices such as the American Republican party.

Contrary to the atmosphere of the Executive Board, the Advisory Committee on Administrative and Budgetary Questions (ACABQ), exhibited a different approach. During its many years of operation, ACABQ was chaired by a Tanzanian, renowned for his probing questions. He had served the UN for 38 years and later authored a book titled, "The Anatomy of Decay: A United Nations Memoir." Like other long-serving, New York-based UN staff, he justified his on-going chairmanship as essential to safeguarding the budgets of the United Nations and all its agencies. The ACABQ oversaw promotions of UN employees, the creation of new posts and the establishment of pay grades.

---

[8]General Assembly resolution 48/162 of 20 December 1993 created the Executive Board, which consists of representatives from 36 countries who serve on a rotating basis. The Board provides intergovernmental support and supervision for the activities of UNDP, UNFPA, and UNOPS in accordance with the policy guidance of the General Assembly, the Economic and Social Council, and the United Nations Charter.

Taken together, these initial experiences were not propitious. However, three months after I arrived in New York, my wife and son joined me from China. Our accommodation and schooling challenges were settled and I began to calm down and look more positively at the prospect of living and working in New York. It was spring. I revelled in the early morning walk to the office. My senses were alert to shops being opened, hearing the accents, seeing the wares being displayed on the street, the flowers for sale in buckets, the smells of a beginning day. Rather than looking at my feet, I looked up to discover the New York architecture. I was taking it all in. For the first time, I felt that I was now a UN official![9] With my growing confidence and in the absence of any briefing, I was keen to research the best practices in other parts of the UN system.

Opportunities for dialogue presented themselves at the regular meetings of the UN HR fraternity. Attendees were mostly Europeans, Canadians, Americans, and Australians although, having spent so many years in the field I still felt like an outsider. This group represented an in-crowd raised within the system, skilled in its manoeuvres and comfortable with their protected presence in their respective European headquarters. They formed a clique who met regularly and knew their way around the language, acronyms and lifestyle associated with their privilege. Although I never felt part of the group, my experience serving in various field posts enabled me to contribute from a different perspective particularly in discussions around the transitional and changing nature of the workplace.

After this "settling-in" period, my immediate concern focussed on staff/management relationship. Of necessity, it was one step at a time beginning at the 'ground floor' level. Partly by design, partly by instinct I began to improvise an HR strategy. Though not always easy, my extensive meetings with staff members began to produce results. While branch chiefs would often bury themselves in other commitments or meetings, a not uncommon way to avoid tough HR decisions, staff were soon lining up at my door and telling me their stories. Such was the acceleration in personal contact and email communication I began to devote 5 till 7 o'clock each afternoon to responding.

Upper management was not entirely to blame for the grim atmosphere. There were many who strived to contribute towards what was clearly

---

[9]Later, I engaged a consultant to write an introductory guide for those transferring to New York. This followed the experience of our new Executive Director who wanting to shop at the Ikea store, paid hundreds of dollars to a taxi to take her to New Jersey not knowing that Ikea provided a free daily 'courtesy' bus from Penn Station.

important within our mission-focused organisation. That said, a review undertaken in 2002 confirmed that the UNFPA management culture was driven by a top-down approach. The report found "top management dominated decision-making, intimidated staff, and triggered a mindset that was extremely risk-averse."[10] In cases where staff members had relevant experience, they were rarely consulted. In my case, I was never once approached for comment on any aspect of our China strategy despite the fact that I had just spent 5 years in charge of the Beijing office. It was a silo structure, with little lateral interaction or discussion of operational issues among branches and divisions.

Contrary to expectation, I found many HQ staff preferred to stay permanently in New York and find ways to undermine the rotation exercise. Among the litany of reasons for not moving to the 'field' was their desire not to jeopardise residential eligibility for a green card. To this end they would come up with excuses such as house mortgages, children's schooling, care of elderly parents or perhaps their spouse's indispensable role with their NY government mission. While these excuses may have been perfectly genuine and reasonable in any other context, they did not accord with the UNFPA employment mandate that prided itself on being a field-based organisation.[11] For those who did agree to move out of New York, particularly long-serving general service staff who sought temporary change, a three-month field assignment was an acceptable way of breaking the routine. This worked very well for some, even when transferred to hardship stations such as Liberia and Afghanistan.

Over the next seven years in HR, I became exposed to the underbelly of the organisation. As HR chief I was privy to personal aspects of the lives of staff that some may have preferred to keep private. I dealt with matters such as armed robbery, house break-ins, tropical illnesses, substance abuse, rapes, and death. There were institutional crises of staff mistreatment, inappropriate behaviour, minor corruption, and misuse of office assets including vehicles and equipment. Such cases required me to investigate and provide counselling. To establish the authenticity of claims I insisted on three independent sources confirming the truth or otherwise. I was at pains to let staff know that I was available to listen, that whatever they told me I would treat

---

[10]Management review of the Division for Management Services, HRSolutions, 2002.

[11]In the 2017/2018 Reform Agenda it was proposed that 17 posts from the Technical Division be moved to the field. Whether the occupants of these posts actually went remains a moot point. As had happened so often in the past many of the posts were unfilled or where they were the staff member would simply declare they were unable or unwilling to make the move.

in the strictest confidence and that I would endeavour to propose a constructive solution to their dilemma. In so doing, I accepted that you came to know more about staff members than you would like to know, or that they would like you to know. While I might be able to provide valuable assistance to a staff member, I always ran the risk of incurring their later resentment. They did not always want to be reminded or to know that you knew.

It was my firm belief that training opportunities were imperative in helping staff meet expectations and their understanding of the HR role. We had a budget allowing the newly formed training and development branch to assume responsibility for upgrading staff skills and to this end we began publishing an OHR newsletter titled "Amina".[12] Publicly, the EC set great store on training programmes, lauding their commitment to "expanding the skills of the workforce." However, at the mere mention of a crisis in the organisation's larger budget, training and development expenditure was the first to be cut. This ensured under-spending despite being spoken of as an essential need.[13] Nonetheless, in response to demand we were able to continue our focus on management training, substantive team-building exercises and online technical courses.

Unlike the private sector, staff employment at the UN is often of long duration. The benefits of the education grant and pension fund are attractive and not to be given up lightly. Early on, I was surprised to find that more than 55% of the professional workforce in UNFPA was over 50[14] with most having served for more than ten years. Contrary to practice in much of the private sector most staff at HQ had worked in the same positions with little variation in tasks since their initial appointment. There was very little turnover.[15] In common with other multinational organisations, there were also loose groupings around individuals, relationships with an ED past or present, and enduring friendships.

When I became aware of these clusters I began to recognize it was not senior management alone that perpetuated the oppressive atmosphere. One of the earliest issues I had to deal with were the complaints of general service staff that, in addition to the other groupings, nationalities were so dominating a branch that qualified outsiders were being excluded. I wondered if this was the norm or the exception? On examination, although incidents certainly

---

[12]Named after one of the plays we wrote all those years ago in Bangladesh: "Amina's Road to Happiness".

[13]Globally, comparable organisations to the UN spend 5–6% on training, the UN spends 1.25%.

[14]During my time at headquarters, 94 out of 168 Professional staff were over 50 and 50% of the general service staff were likewise.

[15]Later, I saw how the UN was for some, not only a career opportunity but also (and contrary to UN rules), a means to gain permanent residency in the United States.

did occur, I concluded they were the exception rather than the rule. From my experience at HQ most staff, irrespective of nationality, were engaged in and earnestly tackling their assignments. The mix of nationalities working at the UN is one of the great virtues of the system, perhaps because most were western-educated with English as the common language.

Of course, as any HR practitioner will tell you, there are always going to be staff who want you to massage the rules to suit their own situation. What was troublesome in UNFPA and of course applied elsewhere, was the apparent reluctance of managers to convey bad news, especially when calling for improved performance from a staff member. They much preferred to be the conveyor of only good news. This attitude prevailed when dealing directly with a staff member but more particularly in their written performance assessment which were, inevitably, positive, even glowing. I wondered, why.

Such fear on the part of managers was not unfounded as staff realised that if they had an ED willing to listen to their situation, they could leapfrog over their supervisor in the hope of achieving a favourable outcome. As a result, managers stopped making personnel decisions knowing they were not always the final arbiter. With the chain of accountability broken, OHR was forced to act as manager rather than facilitator of staff movement and promotions. We should have been the last port of call in a dispute but we were often criticised if we did intervene or again if we did not. Whether it was at HQ, a regional or country office, the organisational culture was largely individually driven and determined by the respective directors.

I endeavoured to add some fairness into performance assessments by maintaining an historical record on every staff member. While this met with partial success only in very difficult cases was remedial action taken.[16] Poor performers continued to be tolerated, compensated or moved elsewhere with a glowing reference. Later I came to see that this typified general UN practice.

Clearly, the formal appraisal system was a failure, a whitewash. Personnel decisions were being made on the basis of corridor gossip, the views of the division director and the judgment of the ED. These practices contradicted the mandate that defined HR procedures and the need for transparency. My head was reeling. HR was the only office answerable to both the ED and the staff. If you did things by the book you were considered disparaging and needlessly bureaucratic. In contrast, acting at the whim of the executive

---

[16]In the view of a staff member who worked with UNFPA in the 1980's, about one quarter of the HQs staff were not suitable for the job they had been hired for. The question then became what to do with them? The retiree explained that the then ED put the obvious "dead-wood" in a separate unit called Policy and Development where they produced a book each year that the retiree said nobody read. But, they were occupied and out of the way of others doing their job!

director made you appear little more than a mouthpiece. It was a lose/lose situation. I felt as if I were skimming over the top, uncertain of my own insight or authority, dependant on the information my HR staff presented to me. This was unsettling because I needed to be able to speak with authority across a range of subjects yet simply didn't feel confident to do so.

To help me address what I perceived as shortcomings in our system I opted to attend management training. This was held at a centre close to Times Square where I found myself in the company of staff from organisations as diverse as Taco Bell, the defence industry and local government. The participants were young, smart, and eager. To my surprise, the Taco Bell people publicly declared their commitment to their employees with an eloquence and moral authority that out-matched anything I had heard at the UN. Later, as part of my education in best practices, I attended an HR conference in Las Vegas along with fifteen thousand other professionals. I was astonished at the scale of the industry and its ancillary offshoots. I recorded everything I heard, ranging from competency assessments, psychological techniques, interview processes, performance appraisals to acceleration pools. When I reported back to the EC, they listened with interest but then moved on to the next agenda item. They felt the UN was different.

In my HQ interviews and introductory branch meetings, a common theme that emerged was a perceived lack of challenge among staff members. Rightly or wrongly, they felt their tasks were mundane and routine. They had not joined the UN for this kind of monotony. For the general staff they also felt 'stuck', unable to make the transition to the professional ranks. Despite applying for new positions, managers often left them in the dark about why they had not succeeded. I had already ascertained that their personnel record would neither record shortcomings nor constructive comment. Line managers tended not to have a frank exchange with staff. Increasingly, I saw this behaviour as typifying not only the UNFPA but the UN system.

Despite their frustration I saw that leaving the organisation was not an option for many staff. They stood to lose too much. The conundrum they faced was described by a close colleague:

Every person who goes to work for the UN remembers their first day. They were proud, drawn to and inspired by the mission. The institution then spends the next 10 years hammering that out of them! People either become stuck or complacent, begrudgingly staying with the institution, their ed grants, their pension, into their old age and contributing to what can be a stale working environment.[17]

---

[17] Personal interview.

From my experience, was this a valid criticism? I knew we had an aging work force and that employment at the UN was mostly lengthy but could be short and sharp. I also knew that, for many, despite their initial rationale for joining the UN, their dependence on the education grant and pension fund assumed priority. Then there were others who imbued with idealism but constrained by the heaviness of the UN bureaucracy, tended to leave before their commitment evolved into frustration or cynicism. The latter was most apparent with young recruits who despite their lifelong dream to work at the UN, ended up handling files which management thought below their senior level. The recruit would come to me disheartened by the routine nature of their administrative roles. They would tell me how they prepared material for their managers only to receive no recognition. Not infrequently did I then see these talented but frustrated performers seek positions in the World Bank, the NGOs, and the universities. On the other hand, there were those who had worked conscientiously for years in the same job and appeared comfortable in positions that offered no challenges or opportunities to expand their abilities.

Many staff complaints encompassed the view of themselves as being either underemployed, over employed or employed incorrectly, grudgingly accepting tasks not defined in their job descriptions. If an issue arose, managers would justify their instruction by pointing to the standard final task in the job description, "…other duties as directed".

I decided that one way to address conflict of interest issues was to look at what people were actually doing and to conduct an analysis of workloads. But how to do that? Re-grading a post, upwards or downwards or keeping it at the same level, required all-party agreement and an independent assessment. But living with the results could be difficult with major implications for the staff concerned. A close colleague once referred to classification as the sledgehammer of HR management.

Any efforts to reform the recruitment and promotion system were often met by fierce determination of senior staff to maintain the status quo. This persistent attitude presented the now renamed DHR with the greatest challenge to job classification reform. The more we thought about it the more we came to the view that we needed to restructure, in part to also remind staff that their job belonged to the organisation, not them. Put simply: did we need a differently shaped organisation and if so, did we have the best people to match the roles we wanted? Would our mandate then remain the same? "Reengineering" became the buzzword and from there the "Workforce Planning Exercise" (WFPE) was launched. It ran for 18 months.

The WFPE was an initiative to determine what organisational restructuring was required. More fundamentally, we were questioning the ongoing relevance of our mandate and whether or not staff abilities and qualifications matched the organisation we wanted. What was unknown, however, was what the ED wanted, and would she be prepared to countenance the changes called for. We hoped the outcomes of the WFPE would empower rather than disparage staff.

Headquarters staff were optimistic, but we were cautious because reengineering implied openness, self-examination, and a preparedness to change. We began by asking people to write down what they actually did during office hours. We anticipated how they spent their time would be inconsistent with their job descriptions. We also suspected staff were performing tasks that did not equate with their knowledge and skills.

Alongside the WFPE initiative, we launched a field-based staff survey to determine the impact of operational challenges at headquarters. As a result, a reorientation of goals, strategy, process and tools to support a new structure was proposed. Particular emphasis was placed on field representatives being held accountable for managing and delivering the mandate. Cost-effective country programmes were, after all, the primary goal of UNFPA. Who were we at headquarters to get in the way of our field offices delivering life-saving programmes?

We invited senior management to a retreat (November 1999) to redress UNFPA goals and objectives. There was an infectious enthusiasm, a buzz that suggested the potential for genuine transformation. Sure, the discussion was based on the corporate language often heard at the UN; about how we wanted to make the organisation "results-based," capable of "self-monitoring and evaluation" and "cementing linkages within and between organisational units both at headquarters and in the field." But the momentum was there. Everybody agreed urgent change was required. Whilst the retreat was a defining moment, we still knew that implementing change would be challenging precisely because it would require participatory consensus to translate findings into practice. We anticipated that would be uncomfortable because the basic assumption was that we needed a smaller headquarters and an enhanced field presence. Fairly monumental changes were envisioned.

To address this reality, we established the "Action Coordination Teams". In accord with its specific acronym, each ACT was required to assess and propose mid-term and long-term implementation plans ("doables"). We were inundated with ideas. The place was buzzing with proposals.

The teams debated our strategic focus, UNFPA's corporate identity, knowledge networking and information systems, development and management of human resources and field office needs. It was an exercise in lateral thinking, with people energetically debating a whole range of options around redeployment, redistribution, reengineering, downsizing, outsourcing, and telecommuting. Staff frustrations were addressed, and younger staff involved. It was agreed that the field must be empowered, and representatives held accountable. There was a sense that the administration had put itself on the line.

When the six ACTs plans were finally in place, they were considered by a Change Support Group (CSG) consisting of senior management. Colleagues were still urging caution against trying to flip the organisational pyramid. We were advised to be more realistic than utopian in our thinking. Undaunted, we forged ahead. By the time of the global meeting (15–18 May 2000), the CSG had agreed on 107 recommendations including the transfer of posts to the field. Going well beyond an abstract exploration of reform was an action plan of immediate "doables", followed by mid- and longer-term goals. With the final WFPE report now in we awaited the announcement of new measures at the upcoming global meeting.

The chair of the CSG made the presentation at that meeting. The staff waited expectantly for the announcement of the WFPE outcomes. But where was the executive director? She was not in the meeting. I found her at work in her office. I reminded her that this was a critical moment in the proceedings and that one of her division directors had declared "The water was rising." Rapidly we moved to the plenary for her announcement but to our puzzlement she insisted that organisational arrangements remained the prerogative of senior management. This was followed by the decision that the proposal to establish regional offices would be shelved. To cap it off, instead of the substantial number of proposed posts for transfer to the field, only two would move from headquarters. The bubble had burst. I had witnessed the power of an executive director, as the final arbiter of decisions made within an entrenched hierarchy. The lesson learnt was that authority at the top would not only continue to define the organisation but also determine its functioning and atmosphere. During my seven years in New York it would be the management style of the ED who would prescribe the working environment.

My experience with reform during these years at HQ set me to thinking about leadership in the UN system; about the cast of characters who seemed to set a tone determined by their view of the world. The system was extremely hierarchical on the one hand, yet on the other loathe to interfere with the performance of management staff other than moving them upwards or side-ways. Why did staff publicly fall into line with management directives while consistently complaining in the corridors. After all, they didn't have much to lose by challenging the status quo, their contracts were certainly not going to be terminated. Transfer to the field was possible but in my mind that was not such a bad outcome. We were, after all, a field-based organisation. Was it simply a fear of change, or did it have to do with maintaining a post at headquarters and its accompanying benefits?[18]

As a consequence, HQ seemed rarely to be viewed by country offices in a positive light, often blamed for every complaint no matter how trivial. One way to address this situation, or so I thought, was to refer to trip reports written by division directors when they travelled to the field, a mandatory requirement to facilitate follow-up action. Of particular importance from a DHR perspective was that the EC become aware of the divisional directors' observations and recommendations. I hoped this would provide a useful and productive sense of the realities on the ground. It was a forlorn hope. As I discovered, the geographic division directors rarely submitted reports. This meant we were often surprised when verbal complaints reached us from field staff. It led to the question of what was actually achieved on these very frequent visits by division directors.[19]

So it fell to DHR, or, more specifically, me, to visit troubled field offices. I travelled often, charged with sorting out dysfunctional staff management relationships and to encouraging what was euphemistically referred to as "teambuilding." Quickly it became apparent that, contrary to the stated best practices of the UN, some staff were vulnerable to exploitation from an informal power structure. I found that the origin for these office breakdowns was threefold. First, a long-serving national officer who was challenged by or took exception to a new country representative. Second, young, idealistic, and ambitious international staff being either ignored or, alternatively, finding themselves favoured by international staff over and above the nationals. They could also find themselves struggling with the attitudes of long-serving national staff who were locally seen as the UNFPA office (e.g., "internationals come and go but we are always here and always will be"). The third reason had to do with the behaviour of the representative themselves and their approach. Fortunately, these incidents were few but at times they were

---

[18]Notably the education grant and the future pension fund.

[19]Later, when I took up my assignment in Viet Nam, I made it a requirement that any staff member visiting from the Bangkok regional office or from headquarters met with all the staff and briefed them and that, on their return, sent us a copy of their trip report. We succeeded with the briefing but very rarely with the report.

sufficiently concerning that they threatened to bring the organisation into disrepute.

Whether it was Zimbabwe, Uzbekistan, Haiti, Zambia, Jamaica, Slovakia, Turkey, Jordan, Sri Lanka or elsewhere, my 'missions' from headquarters did identify a 'cult of personality' embedded in the leadership structure. Typically, the complainant would approach DHR verbally or by email to declare unfair treatment of some kind to the point that their relationship with the representative or supervisor had broken down. Allegations might point to the representative having favourites amongst the staff, or expecting staff to attend to their personal needs. Perhaps the complaint might be about exploitation of entitlements or misuse of programme funds. Interestingly, accusations never came to our attention via the responsible director of the concerned geographic division who was regularly travelling to the region from New York, but directly from the affected country office staff.

Similarly at HQ, I continued to find that many supervisors avoided direct involvement in staff disputes despite this being one of their key management responsibilities. We couldn't break the pattern where staff empowerment ultimately came with access to the ED on the 19th floor. This shortcoming meant that individual complaints dragged on, with the same disgruntled staff member seeking a meeting with me again and again. They could sense when management was unhappy with them, after all there was gossip in the corridors, but they never received any constructive criticism face-to-face, just compliments or generalisations that the problem lay elsewhere. This was compounded by a lack of continuity in decision making and an absence of good records.

On and on went the trend to report all staff achievements in their annual performance reviews as 'exceptional',[20] irrespective of reality or whether they were simply delivering their normal and expected outputs. With everyone achieving "more than expected" measurements it became clear they were based on behaviour and personal relationships, not results. This ran the risk of promoting poor performers to more senior levels by virtue of their positive performance rating.

Performance assessments were made more difficult when I realised that higher level staff were sometimes unwilling to undertake base-level tasks nor, in many instances, the required technical work.[21] This resulted in the appointment of temporary employees to deal with the overflow of mundane

---

[20]The highest possible grading in the Performance Appraisal Review. Followed by 'fully achieved', 'partially achieved', and 'did not achieve outputs'. (New PAR).

[21]"I am an accountant as well as a demographer. I am not a clerk!" This was particularly noticeable in the management services area.

work as well as, surprisingly, the common practice of employing consultants to complete tasks that were listed as part of a professional's job description. Together, these practices, when coupled with the extraordinarily long and cumbersome recruiting and hiring process, impeded the development of effective teams.

One-way of DHR addressing these shortcomings was to routinely remind managers of what they had said earlier or what had been discussed in management meetings. The problem was that verbal exchanges and decisions were rarely officially recorded. For this reason I became even more addicted than ever to keeping my own notes during performance appraisal meetings.

Our major challenge then became one of how to re-position an organisation with an uneven and top heavy management to staff ratio. What to do? I flew to Pittsburgh where I learnt about competency assessment methods. On this basis, we began to engage in performance planning that involved review by peers, mid and end-year appraisals and identifying training needs aligned with career aspirations. Numeric ratings by supervisors were discontinued, replaced by corporate language denoting levels of proficiency. All of these changes were accepted by the Executive Committee, but when it came to including a record of the number of times a country representative actually left the capital to visit rural-based projects, where the bulk of the population lived, it was considered a step too far.

During my years in HR I found the sustained negativity about the organisation from certain sources a pitfall to be avoided. Overwhelmingly, it was important to appreciate that most of the staff were good people working hard to make a difference. But, after being briefed by many of my colleagues within the UN system, a common picture began to emerge that depicted an excess of higher-level professionals,[22] and senior general service staff, over those in the lower ranks.[23] This resulted in an excessive burdening of junior staff expected to undertake duties beyond their official level of responsibilities. There appeared to be a lack of transparency in the initial recruitment process whereby the pool of candidates tended to be weighted in favour of internal applicants including those from within the wider UN system. Moreover, the number of unfilled positions never seemed to diminish, with some deliberately kept open pending the availability of a preferred candidate. In

---

[22]In the 'common system' of the UN civil service, "… there are five levels of professional posts (P1 to P5) to which appointments and promotions are supposedly, but in reality, far from universally, made on merit alone. Immediately above, in ascending order of rank are Directors D1 and D2. Assistant Secretary-General and Under Secretary-General. The Executive Director of WFP (and UNFPA) is at the Under-Secretary General/Deputy Director-General level". Ingram op cit p. 8.

[23]G1 and G7's—locally recruited staff with 1–7 years of work experience.

my view and to offset these realities, we needed to look again at the benefits of decentralization.

Of necessity, this would require a redesign of country offices including the regionally based country support teams (CSTs) and importantly, a change in the approach of headquarters. To this end, fourteen country offices were visited by 30 staff divided into teams each with specific terms of reference. Their findings confirmed that field offices operated in markedly different ways, that there was no standard structure. In brief, our challenge became one of identifying some key inputs that might better determine operational efficiency and consistency.

This led to the introduction of new word into the UN lexicon, 'Typology'. In a circular distributed on 12 July 2002, the Executive Director said:

> ... The introduction of a staffing typology based on demonstrable programme needs offers tremendous opportunities for the strategic realignment of our country offices. It is intended to help UNFPA move away from a sometimes ad hoc and unsystematic approach to assigning staff strength and determining office size in countries, to a more objective and coherent system that sets for standards for country office capacities in different countries. At the same time, the system maintains some flexibility for UNFPA to take strategic considerations into account when determining its presence at the country level. Overall, the new staffing patterns call for additional posts and a strengthened field presence, and we are including the necessary funds to reflect these changes in the revised 2002–2003 biennial budget.

The typology programme called for a new staffing pattern including the additional post of "operation manager" seened as needed to strengthen the Fund's field presence. The budget to do this would come following a reduction in positions at HQ. For this senior managers would need to remodel their behaviour, to be more effective with less. The words were new, but the ideas were a product of those earlier ACTs which I had introduced during my first tilt at reform.[24] The difference now was the support of the new ED who agreed there was a fundamental problem with the organisational structure and that it could only change if there was a change in the behaviour of people.

The "Typology Implementation Guide"[25] informed field office staff about the exercise. Starting with the specifics of a country programme, offices were required to review current posts, determine what was necessary, and what was not, and then match staff to requirement. If superfluous, redundancies

---

[24] 1998–2001.
[25] 140 pages.

were offered. Where vacancies appeared, new staff recruited. This also applied to the 85 members of the CSTs who were required to resign and reapply for their regional office advisor positions. Geographic locations had to be taken into account. For example, Latin America clearly had different needs to Africa. Throughout the process we interviewed over one hundred field staff. From there it required considerable effort to devise a process that would encompass advertising posts, screening applicants, shortlisting, interviewing, and appointing and designing redundancy packages. Were there winners and losers in these lengthy and substantial exercises? True to UN form, virtually everyone was accommodated.

It is my view that the success of an organisation such as UNFPA is contingent on strong and fair leadership. A consultative, inclusive ED with trust in their directors encourages robust discussions with potential for consensus. An authoritarian ED who prefers to ignore DHR recommendations and rides roughshod over alternative opinions reduces the HR management team to a mere cypher.[26] Critically, I felt that after spending seven years in DHR, changes at the bottom levels continued to be dependent on action taken at the top. Where these were absent my confidence in the system waned. Perhaps I knew too much about too many people. Certainly, I had witnessed the underbelly of the organisation.

At this point the ED suggested I stay on in New York but in a different role. However, I decided enough was enough. Better to return to the field where I was confident from past experience, of the potential to make a real and tangible difference. Better to be part of a distinctive UN country team, at the front line of development, rather than a daily commuter to a midtown skyscraper. It was time to restore my faith in the UN system and reverse the slide into cynicism only too common among HR professionals. Thus, despite my pride in my loyal group of DHR colleagues and all we had achieved, not to mention sadness to be foregoing all the cultural and other excitements that the "Big Apple" had to offer, Viet Nam beckoned.

---

[26]A reality experienced by one of my successors who told me that during the regular two-hour Monday morning meeting, the ED (who was not one I worked with) made all the decisions irrespective of the recommendations agreed to by the HR professionals or any in-house advisory committee.

10

No More Business as Usual: Viet Nam

"You can't solve current problems with current thinking...current problems are the result of current thinking" Albert Einstein[1]

"You're looking much better" declared the Vice-Minister for the Population, Family and Children Commission (PFCC). I thanked him, presuming this was an expression of Vietnamese courtesy. "No, you are!" he insisted when I looked sceptical. How could this be? I had only been in the country for two weeks and here was someone commenting on my appearance. I looked in the mirror. I could not see any difference but when others expressed the same view, I had to assume that, yes, being out of the bubble of headquarters had made a difference. I felt better and my face showed it. The improvement had begun at the airport. On arrival in Ha Noi[2] we were delighted to be greeted by a local staff member the moment we exited the plane and walked into the terminal. There she was, holding a sign. Wonderful! This was very promising. But, hold on, there was a hiccup. Where were the Vietnamese visas for my wife and son?[3] "No worries," my welcoming colleague declared, "A minor detail. I'll handle it." We sat and waited, watching as our new "fixer"

---

[1] As quoted to me by a senior Vietnamese government official.

[2] In Vietnamese, 'Việt' refers to the region that covers Viet Nam to the North, and 'Nam' refers to the South, so together Việt Nam represents the whole country. Often this is anglicised into Vietnam, when really the word should be separated into two: Viet Nam. The same goes for Ha Noi, and so on.

[3] He was joining us to fill in the six months between the end of the Northern Hemisphere school year before joining his sister for the new university year in Australia.

© The Author(s), under exclusive license to Springer Nature Switzerland AG 2021
I. Howie, *Reflections on a United Nations' Career*, Springer Biographies, https://doi.org/10.1007/978-3-030-77063-1_10

went from official to official, all of whom she knew, and had the pages of the concerned passports appropriately stamped. Then she delivered the forms to us, we filled them in, and, in no time, were legally admitted. Not quite the bureaucracy we anticipated in this one-party state.

Outside, in the car park, we met the senior UNFPA driver, a tall, dignified man of few words. We shook hands and together put the luggage in the boot. Over time, I came to know this colleague well. On this, our first drive into the city, with our son sitting between us, he pointed out the sights. Excitedly we looked this way and that, viewing a rural landscape that during our years in the country would change to high rise suburbs. Multiple trips later I was still engrossed with what I saw, the only difference being the phone calls I now made announcing that I had landed and would be home soon. Extraordinary, really, the mental navigation one makes from the newness of first arrival to the everyday familiarity of the routine. You arrive knowing no-one, having never been there before, and in no time a trip to the airport becomes pedestrian. While these re-assignments never came naturally to me, over time I learnt to make the transitions. It was the family support that mattered and, soon after arrival in Ha Noi, we were moving out of temporary hotel accommodation into what became our permanent home. Located on Thanh Nien Road, it was an apartment block situated on a narrow strip between two lakes—Chuc Bach[4] and Tay Ho (West Lake).

Now settled I was eager to meet the UNFPA staff and get to know them. From experience, I knew that when a new representative took up their appointment, they inherited staff rather than recruited them. So it was with the Viet Nam team who I came to know well in the coming months. In what was the most inclusive office I worked in, they were a joy. Not only did we work together but lunched together, every day. And when we travelled, we travelled as a team. There were eight members covered by the office budget and another twenty-two financed by the current country programme, the Sixth, 2001–2005.[5] Included were a mix of professional and general service

---

[4] A 'must see' for the American visitor (not so the Vietnamese) because it was into this lake that US Senator and Presidential candidate, John McCain, ditched his plane during the Viet Nam War. What mattered to the Vietnamese was the Tran Quoc Pagoda also located in walking distance of our apartment. This was the oldest of its kind in Ha Noi, dating back to the 6th century during the reign of Emperor Ly Nam De Dynasty (544–548). Situated on a small peninsula in Tay Ho, visitors flocked there escaping for a moment the noise and traffic of nearby Thanh Nien Road.

[5] In 2004 the World Bank was the biggest donor to the Vietnamese health sector followed by Japan, the European Union, Sweden, Luxembourg, and Australia. Approximately USD1 billion ODA was provided with a third being concessional loans mostly to upgrade hospitals. These donors along with the Dutch and New Zealand governments were also important contributors to UNFPA programmes both its Sixth, US27 million in total and then its Seventh, 2006–2010, US$28 million.

staff and apart from myself and five others, all were Vietnamese. Standard UN job classifications applied—assistant representative, programme officer, programme associate, project officer, admin and finance officer, secretary, UN Volunteer, and intern. Given the nature of the government, it was not surprising that the older members had strong connections to the administration. A number had previously worked for the General Statistics Office (the GSO) with whom our office collaborated on population data. They often recalled the 'American War'[6] and their evacuation as students to the mountains or to Eastern Europe. Now, after many years working with UNFPA, they were part of an affluent middle class with aspirations far beyond their proletariat upbringing. Most were out-of-touch with the rural and working-class masses whose needs they were to champion. Understandably, they saw UN employment as providing a standard of living well above the average. Newer appointees were younger. Following a relaxation of the requirement that staff come from government,[7] they were more likely to be chosen on merit. While they came from comparable backgrounds to their seniors, being newer they had been exposed to western ideas and spoke fondly of their time studying abroad.[8] One thing I learned quickly from them was how they often felt 'bogged down' in project details.[9] Additionally, despite many having completed post-graduate studies in English, no mean feat, when it came to analysis they would often struggle. This meant I spent a great deal of time discussing with them what they really wanted to say and re-writing their communiques. Was this preoccupation of mine with English clarity important in the scheme of things? Probably not, and I was careful not to make it an issue, especially when it came to electronic communication. I also recalled how a representative could favour international staff, no matter how young or temporary their appointments, simply because they spoke English and had a cultural link. Quite rightly, national staff resented this, and I had no desire to go down the same path.

---

[6] The Vietnam War as it known in the West, 1962–1975, saw many Vietnamese children relocated out of the cities to the mountains or to Eastern Europe. Colleagues would tell me you could guess where the child had gone by the height and build of the older person. Poor nutrition in the highlands or the richer one out of the country.

[7] This situation exactly mirrored the staffing profile found in China, Mongolia and DPRK—all one-party states. A previous UN Resident Coordinator to Viet Nam had negotiated direct recruitment in 1994.

[8] But such is the hold of the pension that most of the staff (national and international) stay with the UN for most of their working lives.

[9] Understandable when you consider that government project staff did not work full-time on our UNFPA funded projects. They had their ongoing normal duties. Consequently, UNFPA staff had to fill in the void.

There was a good mix of skills among the staff. There were those who operated well at field level and did so because they spoke the local language and had provincial contacts. There were also those who were more successful in an office environment because they could work through the detail, had the capacity to see trends over time, and could deal one-on-one with senior government officials (often their old colleagues). But where many struggled was in dealing with youth projects. Unlike most Vietnamese young people most of our staff had never been to a disco or 'hung out' in bars.[10] Being among the 5% who had gone to university (at that time), they were intently focused on the schooling of their own children, and saving to send them overseas.

Among my other first impressions was how the international Junior Programme Officers (JPOs) were being under-utilised. By its very nature, the JPO position is intended to be a learning experience and, as such, requires careful supervision and training. JPOs are not just an occupant of a seat but expect to make a meaningful contribution. On meeting with them I heard how their experiences tended to follow a common path. While mixing well they still had to write their own terms of references and were often given random tasks. Not surprisingly, this meant they had to find their own way as best they could (despite the culture shock, language difficulties and uncertainties about who they could speak to).[11] Left to work independently meant not being invited to meetings. Not wanting to create an artificial division, I saw this needed to change. So, I began meeting regularly with the JPO's and the interns, ensured they had an external representative role according to their specialisation, linked them one-on-one with a senior local officer and initiated monthly team meetings inclusive of everyone.

Experience had also taught me not to rush any changes, but to quietly observe and listen. Quickly I learnt how Viet Nam was made up of 58 centrally controlled provinces, which were then divided into provincial cities

---

[10]In 2004, 20% of total pregnancies were before nineteen years of age (Youth Union statistic) but when I tried to have condoms distributed in bars frequented by the young (the 'hot spots' as they were referred to), I was told this was not possible because the venues would then be thought of as 'social evils', condoms being associated with commercial sex work. Surprisingly, however, the Women's' Union distributed its own brand of condom under the commercial name of "Hello". Although, with 26% of commercial condoms in Ha Noi and Ho Chi Minh City found to be substandard (UNFPA Report 2014), condom use was not always reliable.

[11]Illustrative of the challenges JPO's faced was the following experience. "I was the first of three to arrive in 2003. There were no scheduled meetings, only quick introductions, no explanation of the administrative arrangements and no clarity of what was to be done and where to find things. Three of us had the same terms of reference but we were not included in the office organigram. We had to find something to do. Yes, we were integrated socially but not professionally. Local staff simply didn't understand how difficult it was for a newcomer to find a role." Meeting with interns and JPO's, July 2005, Notebook #4.

and rural districts, which in turn were divided into towns and communes. Occupation by the Chinese for a thousand years, had left its legacy as evidenced in Chinese languages signs, Buddhist shrines, art, and a Confucian way of life. Often overlooked by the visitor was the Chinese demographic footprint, with settlement by large numbers of ethnic Han Chinese.

I knew that the country had faced many hardships, not least of which was the independence struggle with the French (the Indo-China War, 1946–1954), and the 'American War' (1955–1975).[12] Spanning two decades, the American War saw the Catholic South pitted against the Communist North. In 1976 it ended in unification as the Socialist Republic of Viet Nam. The war left the country ravaged, inexperienced in peacetime living and international cooperation, and lacking infrastructure and resources. In the 1970's and early eighties it had followed an economically harmful collectivisation policy. But in 1986 it launched economic reforms known as '*Doi Moi*' (meaning, literally, the 'renovation' of the economy) and opened its doors to international trade. Thereafter, the country moved rapidly from a centrally planned economy to market oriented socialism. Such was the growth that by 2010 it expected to reach middle-income status.

Although having an open economy had helped enormously, the government resolutely continued to conduct its internal affairs as a single-party socialist state under the Communist Party of Viet Nam. During my years living there, the Party maintained tight control and, importantly from the UN's perspective, exercised complete control over the flows and disbursement of foreign aid. My counterparts in the government saw that every project was funnelled through the bureaucracy.

The UNFPA/Viet Nam relationship began in 1977 when the first cooperative programme was launched. At that time, the Fund was the only source of international aid on population issues, a fact the government had not forgotten and for which they were ever grateful.[13] During the decade of the seventies, the country was forecasting a population of 50 million, which was expected to double in the next 30 years. This was spurred on by the long-standing Confucian mentality of "more children more wealth", as well as the fact that family planning facilities, and access to contraceptives, were very poor. As a result, both before and immediately after the war, the average number of children per family was 5, although the government did aim to

---

[12]Three million died in a country of eighteen million. More bombs were dropped per capita than in any other context in history.
[13]Only after 1992 did other donors enter the population field.

reduce this to 2–3.[14] When the war ended the government recognised that the country simply did not have the development capacity to cater to such a large and growing population. With UNFPA's assistance, a decision was made to slow the population growth rate. The focus was on ensuring that all citizens had access to contraception, and that all mothers had the ability to control their fertility. IUD's and the local production of condoms constituted the bulk of the assistance.

The government's efforts in family planning were rewarded in 1999 when Viet Nam received the annual UN Population Award. The citation referred to the fulfilment of the national target of reducing population growth, which in turn contributed to poverty alleviation and the vast improvement of the quality of life of the people. The Total Fertility Rate (TFR) had fallen from 3.8 in 1989 to 2.3 in 1999 (and it continued to fall to 2.12 in 2002), which was considered a great achievement. The UNFPA/Viet Nam relationship had a proud record and rightly so.

Part of this success was due to the 2-child norm that Viet Nam had 'encouraged' since the 1960s in the country's North, and, since the 1970s, in the South. In 1988 this norm was formalised into an official 2-child national policy. Viet Nam had followed the lead of its communist ally China by hoping that a policy of 'later childbearing, longer spacing of children, and fewer children" would be an effective and quick way to slow population growth. A target of 1.7 births per woman was enforced through incentives, including monetary incentives for those having vasectomies and tubal ligations. But punishments were also integral. Meted out for those not following the guidelines were fines (sometimes measured in kilograms of rice), reduced land you received from the commune, increased taxes, higher housing and land rent fees, salary reductions and loss of promotion for government officials, restriction of migration and the forbidding of rural families to move to urban areas. The policy was supported by advertisements, public loudspeaker announcements, and billboards showing a happy one-or-two child family. While the effectiveness of implementation varied from commune to commune, the campaign continued until 1999 when the government slackened the policy and allowed families more freedom in deciding their family size. In 2003 the policy officially ended, and a new policy document, the Population Ordinance (Law), was released. This was great progress for Viet

---

[14]During the war there were no contraceptives. After its conclusion, a family planning movement gradually developed following government's preference for population control. The National Committee for Population and Family Planning (NCPFC) was established in 1987 under the MOH. It began by encouraging two children but with the 1989 census finding a total population of 64 million and a TFR of 3.8, government determined there was a problem. This led to the first population strategy being promulgated in 1990.

Nam, as it represented a major shift in government policy, whereby a key principle of Cairo's ICPD was adhered to, namely, the right of people to decide their own family size. Article 10a of the Ordinance read:

> ...each couple has the right to decide the timing, number, and spacing of births in accordance with their age, health, studies, employment and work, income, and child rearing conditions for every individual and on the basis of the couple's equality.

It was within this social and political context that I arrived in Viet Nam. The Vietnamese government's population goals seemed to align with those of UNFPA. It had recognised the rights' focus.[15] Suggested from the start was that my time in the country would be relatively straightforward. However, soon after we arrived (2004) it became apparent there remained major population issues to be tackled. While conditions had vastly improved since the nineties, many of these improvements had only benefited those living in urban areas. Viet Nam remained an agricultural country with 29% of the population earning less than US$1 a day. Of particular concern were the ethnic minorities who lived in remote and mountainous regions, and were being left behind.[16]

When it came to maternal and reproductive health care, these disparities were hugely visible with those living remotely having considerably less access to the important services. Most babies were born at home, knowledge about reproductive health was low, access to health clinics was poor, there was a lack of health care staff and basic medical equipment, and, due to religious beliefs and community values, the utilisation of existing

---

[15]"We encourage 1 or 2 children through educating couples on how to have a better life but it's their right to have the number they desire." Vice Minister Dat, MPI, briefing an EU/UNFPA delegation, 1 September 2004. Later, at the same briefing, Mdme Thu of the Parliamentary Committee for Social Affairs, explained it this way, "Our population policy since ICPD has been seen as absurd in seeking to limit family size and impose fines. This is why the new ordinance does not limit family size. But this is not to say there is absolute freedom to have whatever number you like. We pay a lot of attention to education, gaps between births and safe deliveries but couples do have the right to decide number and timing while being conscious of their social rights and responsibilities to bring up children properly. There were lots of objections to this ordinance. There are those who say we should not let people decide. Others welcome this freedom. But basically, the latter are those who have single children and want another of the opposite sex plus those who were fined earlier and want a remedy for their suffering." Personal notebook.

[16]Nationally, the poor had the highest rates of 'stunting', were having more children than the wealthier cohorts and completed half as many grades of schooling as their richer counterparts. Population Strategy Workshop, September 2005.

health clinics was minimal.[17] Adding to the challenges was the increasingly imbalanced sex ratio at birth (SRB). As evident in China, India and elsewhere, boys were favoured, girls were not and with HIV/AIDS increasingly prevalent, especially among young people, rural couples were determined to have their boys survive. Not surprisingly, gender equity was also lacking, and the maternal mortality rate (MMR) remained high. Along with internal migration, which was becoming a major issue,[18] these were all challenges highlighted in the 2003 Ordinance towards whose resolution UNFPA was committed to providing the relevant support.

So, it was surprising, that despite these priority development issues, the key population challenge advanced by the government and the media, was the slight rise in the rate of population growth.[19] In the aftermath of the 2003 Ordinance the TFR had grown from 2.12 in 2002 to 2.23. According to the media this was a 'population boom', spurred on by a wave of third births encouraged by the Ordinance's new concept of reproductive rights.[20] Headlines referred to a 'surge' undermining decade of progress in family planning and development. Questions were asked in Parliament about the population increase. Highlighted were the 1.5 million entrants to the labour force each year with only 1 million likely to find employment. A former director of the Viet Nam Ministry for Family Planning and Children (VCFPC) was quoted as saying "the sudden increase in the birth-rate was undermining the country's significant achievements in birth control for the last 10 years." "Particularly concerning," he said, "were the number of families with 3 children increasing by 3% since 2003. Nearly all the accomplishments were being undermined by poor management at every government level. Even local leaders whose wives had given birth for the third time remain at their posts and have not

---

[17]Evidence, my visit to a Commune Health Centre where I was told that ethnic minorities preferred injectable contraception because it did not require a gynaecological examination. "Only husbands can do that."

[18]During my time in Viet Nam the household registration system (hộ khẩu) was still in force. Similar to the Hukou system in China and the Hoju scheme in North Korea, households holding permanent registration (KT1) and migrants within the same district (KT2) had full access to public services. Temporary registration permits (KT3) were granted to other migrants for six to twelve months with the possibility of extension. Migrants who did not possess a household registration book or who were not registered could remain in temporary accommodation for one to three months. KT3 and KT4 households faced higher costs for health, education, water, and electricity. It was under these classifications that 5.5 million people moved between provinces between 1995 and 1999. The outflow was largest from the north central coast (particularly young women migrating to work in the 4,000 factories in the South).

[19]Although we had been forewarned by Mdme Thu. "It is not a population explosion as mentioned in the press. That is sensationalism. It is not at an alarming rate, but Party members have to lead, to set an example and, if not, appropriate measures have to be taken." Meeting with UNFPA's Regional Director, 9 Aug 2005.

[20]The articles often equated fertility with population growth ignoring mortality.

been reprimanded". As a result of the 'crisis', VCPFC was now pushing for an amendment to the Ordinance, one which retracted the 'looser' position on family size conveyed earlier. A third child adds to society's burden, they said. We need to continue setting our targets for every commune and ward.[21] Rights must be associated with duty, it's not anarchy!

My conversations with government officials mirrored VCPFC's concern, and, although the TFR was close to its desired level, it soon became clear that our UNFPA team would be spending much of its time seeking to modify the government's rigid enforcement of its 2-child policy.[22] This was despite the fact that we saw the issues being safe motherhood, improving rural health, adolescent sex and the potentially calamitous sex ratio stemming as it did from the broader gender issues. In anticipation of a crackdown, we decided what was needed now was a scientific study to establish whether or not there had been an acceleration in population growth.

Surprisingly, the initial move came from government. The GSO approached us asking for support to an independent review of the fertility data. While the GSO felt there were no big changes, they were in a 'delicate situation' as they faced increased pressure to justify the draconian action government wanted to take.[23] They now wanted international experts to produce an independent report on what the actual fertility was. I agreed to the necessary funding seeing this as an opportunity to not only discover the facts but, in doing so, present this information to government and, via a series of Vietnamese publications, to the public at large.

We engaged the first of what turned out to be three renowned demographers.[24] The first reviewed population trends, initially from the 2004

---

[21]VCPFC's thousands of population collaborators covered 800 households each throughout the country and they were required to distribute given numbers of IUD's, pills, condoms etc.

[22]I was alerted to this quandary during my initial round of appointments with donors, ambassadors, and senior government ministers. The minister in charge of the Commission for Population, Children and the Family stated that the "...sudden population increase in 2003/2004 was of great concern." Meeting Notes, 11 November 2004. The policy was set nationally but implemented provincially.

[23]Every year in April the GSO undertook a survey on fertility. In January 2005 they were still processing data from April 2004 and had not disseminated any findings. While they felt there were no big changes from the previous year, they were re-appraising the situation being "...in a very difficult situation facing pressure from Government and VCPFC who said their 140,000 field collaborators were reporting a surge. We recognise this is our responsibility but technical assistance from UNFPA would be very helpful" Meeting with GSO, 20 January 2005.

[24]Important to note here is that the Vietnamese did not view UNFPA's Country Support Team (CST) in Bangkok as having the necessary professional skills to undertake the required analysis. They wanted the best with proven international credentials, especially those with recognised publications on Viet Nam. This mirrored broader criticism of the 130 UNFPA staff working globally in CST's and taking a third of the Fund's resources. I recall laughter at a regional meeting of country representatives in Bangkok when told that Objective 1 of the Technical Division at HQ's, who oversaw the CSTs, was to support country offices.

Population Change Survey and, then, subsequent GSO surveys. Found was that there had been a slight increase in the crude rate of natural increase due, most probably, to under-reported mortality rather than an increase in third births. Stressed was the finding that the longer-term trend showed a solid decline in fertility levels, indicating that government and media hype over the population surge, as a result of the Ordinance, was unsubstantiated and did not necessitate a reinstatement of the 2-child policy. In fact, the overwhelming conclusion was that Viet Nam's declining fertility rate over the past 15 years was an 'incontrovertible fact', and that the slight increase in the population in 2004 could not be classified as a population boom. Disappointingly, however, despite our expert analysis, the media continued to demand solutions to the country's apparent uncontrolled and harmful population surge.

So it was that on March 22, 2005, two years after the Ordinance was released, the Politburo of the Central Party introduced Resolution No. 47, titled 'How to Better Promote the Implementation of the Family Planning Policy'. This Resolution not only reaffirmed the birth control strategy,[25] but it requested a revision of the Ordinance insisting there was "…inconsistency in the implementation of the Policy (because of) subjectivism, self-satisfaction of initial achievements, relaxed leadership and guidance, and inconsistency in the implementation of the policy". Called for was a strict enforcement of the two-child policy and punishment of those who did not adhere to it (especially those connected with government in any way). In my efforts to understand this fixation I recalled my experience in China where the State Family Planning Commission deliberately perpetrated a population crisis in order to sustain government funding for their half million size bureaucracy. In Viet Nam, the doctrinaire dictates of a one-party state meant the older, more orthodox, leaders in the National Council on Population, Family, and Children (NCPFC), and in the Viet Nam Family Planning Association (VINAFPA), were not going to give way on the ideological underpinning they had devoted their lives to.

After the publication of Resolution No. 47 we had little choice but to continue our efforts to inform the Party and National Assembly about our concern that the so-called population surge leading to uncontrolled population growth was unwarranted. At a National Workshop organised by the Parliamentary Committee for Social Affairs, I informed the participants (who

---

[25] Resolution 47 stated that "to sustain high economic growth, Viet Nam needs to pursue a population control policy until it has become an industrialized country."

came from the ministries of health and justice, the Office of the Government,[26] and the Viet Nam Fatherland Front[27]) how concerned we were about the decision to revise the Ordinance and potentially reintroduce a one or two child policy. I told them that the focus on numbers and the public administration of family size was questionable, not only from the ICPD perspective, but also because it relegated reproductive health issues to a minor status.[28] That I was able to make the speech was significant. Attested to was both the regard with which the Fund was held but also the discrete and determined way we went about challenging the Government's position. Regrettably, the speech had little effect.[29] We needed to redouble our efforts.

In April 2006, UNFPA and GSO employed the efforts of another demographer to undertake a more comprehensive review of the fertility, mortality, and population growth data from 2000 to 2005. Again, the findings confirmed there was no baby boom, that under-reporting of mortality rates did occur, and that the slight rise in fertility from 2002 to 2003 may have resulted from more couples wanting to have their baby in the 'Year of the Goat', a phenomenon similar to what happened in South Korea.[30]

We again tackled the issue in June 2008 by releasing a publication on population growth prepared by yet another renowned demographer. This third set of findings, confirming the earlier two, was disseminated at a well-attended seminar widely reported in the Vietnamese media. Despite this, the government continued to insist on the need to revise Article 10. As a last resort I drafted a letter for the UN Resident Coordinator (RC) to be sent to the Prime Minister. The letter, delivered on 21 August, conveyed the view that 'based on UNFPA's global experience, the use of penalties to limit family size would not only be counter-productive in achieving population goals, but would also be in contravention of Viet Nam's adherence to the letter and spirit of the ICPD "Programme of Action". Emphasised was that an amendment to Article 10, and the reinstating of non-voluntary family

---

[26]A ministry-level agency made up of multiple departments that assists the government and the Prime Minister to lead, direct and operate government activities.

[27]An umbrella group of mass movements (labour, youth, 'young pioneers') aligned with the Communist Party.

[28]I emphasised that the main focus should be gender equality, uneven access to RH services between those in urban and rural and mountainous areas, the need to improve the quality, choice and availability of sexual and RH services especially for young people, actions to address the HIV/AID epidemic and limited safe motherhood, and the high-level of abortions due to inherent son preference.

[29]Although 37 members of the PCSA rejected VCPFC's request to reverse the 2003 Ordinance and re-introduce the 1 and 2 child policy.

[30]In the Chinese astrological (zodiac) calendar, 2003 was a Year of the Goat. As well as being an animal sign, the symbol was also interpreted as G.O.A.T, the Greatest of All Time. Or the "Golden Goat" as Mdme Thu had called 2003 when she briefed the EU Delegation in September 2004.

planning, was unwelcomed by UNFPA. Regrettably, this letter, much like my earlier speeches, also did not work. The government was going ahead. But we were determined not to give up. On the 15 September, the RC accompanied by the WHO Representative and myself called upon the Minister for Health. Following introductions, the RC, 'in the spirit of partnership', expressed concern about the proposed revision of the Ordinance. In reply, the Minister highlighted the one million babies born every year and the observation being made in the National Assembly that women were having a third child. Any proposed revision to the Ordinance, he said, needed to be in a national context. Why were there so many abortions then,[31] we asked, and wasn't it time, given the country's success in reducing fertility, to move from an administrative approach to one based on the quality of FP services? Do not be too confident about the continuation of a decline, came the reply. "If we do nothing, we will have to face the consequences." A respectful exchange then followed but it was soon clear there was not going to be a change. Later that month, a senior member of the National Assembly told me it was not a question of switching off the brakes, it was about the law and people's responsibilities. The experience of other Asian countries in failing to lift birth rates, once replacement level was exceeded, was not seen as relevant.[32] We were confronted by an impenetrable bureaucracy intent on having its way. On 27 December 2008, the Standing Committee of the National Assembly voted in favour of the revision to the Population Ordinance. Article 10 now read:

> Every couple, every individual has the rights and obligations to implement the campaign on population, family planning and reproductive health care, and to decide the time and spacing of giving birth, having, *một hoặc hai con*, 1 or 2 children.[33]

This was not only a major setback, it also carried with it another issue of concern. The policy rollback was contributing to the uneven sex ratio at birth. More boys were being born than girls owing to human interference and the imbalance was worsening.[34] It was time to move to this new policy challenge.

In common with other Asian countries, especially China and India, there was a clear preference for boys, meaning that female foetuses were either

---

[31] Estimated at more than 2 per woman in her lifetime.

[32] Nor was the GSO data which contradicted that of the MOH. Although there were six provinces where all couples having a third child were penalised, we were told the fault lay with party members, government employees and those working with INGOs accountable to MOFA.

[33] Emphasised is the importance of regulating everything by law.

[34] Nationally 110 to every 100 as against the normal ratio of 105-7 boys to every 100 girls, with the ratio evening out owing to the higher mortality among boys during their first year.

aborted or not registered at birth. This preference was deeply rooted in Viet-namese culture. In part it stemmed from Confucianism, evident in proverbs such as 'Nhất nam viết h˜uu, thập n˜u viết vô', meaning 'one son is having some, ten daughters are having none'. People saw bearing a son as a way to continue the family line, appease one's ancestors, and uphold the family's reputation. Accordingly, Vietnamese women used a range of methods to secure a son including continuing childbearing until a son was born. With the enforcement of the two-child policy, drastic measures were taken including foetal sex determination through ultrasound and, consequently, deliberate abortion of female foetuses. Son preference was a matter of growing concern, particularly the realisation that there was a direct conflict between the pres-sure to bear no more than two children with the equal pressure to produce boys.[35] I now saw it as my goal to communicate these negative synergies to the government, and the population. We used the same approach utilised during the population policy debate only this time we hoped to be more successful. The office compiled all our SRB data, and its analysis, into a new publication. I likened Viet Nam's gender imbalance to that prevailing in China 10 years earlier. Strong male preference paired with government-enforced limited family size. Translated into common usage Vietnamese we disseminated the booklet as widely as we could.[36]

Again the government response was negative. We do not have a problem, they insisted. Sex selection is forbidden by law. Nonetheless there was disagreement between data coming from the GSO and VCPFC with the latter insisting there was no issue. It wasn't until we invited Chinese demog-raphers to brief our counterparts on that country's skewed imbalance that the Government began to recognise the problem and take steps to address it. [37]

Despite these setbacks we continued to work closely and well with our very competent government counterparts. Together we faced challenges common

---

[35] Evidence the following report in the Viet Nam News. 'Lan knew of the Government's policy of two children per family but because she hadn't produced a son, her husband and parents' in-law pressured her to have a third child. "It meant I had violated the government's policy and that my department and I would be fined by hospital leaders so I tried to tighten my pregnancy belt while I was at work so that no-one would know about my situation," said Lan. As it happened, Lan gave birth to a boy. Her entire family was happy, though she personally had lost her monthly bonus and had her salary capped for two years. "I'm happy to have my son but I'm also sad because my department, including my boss, has been fined due to my 'fault'," said Lan'. "Viet Nam encourages two-child families" Viet Nam News, 4 August 2013.

[36] Staff were instructed to distribute the booklets, based on the report, whenever they went to the 'field' thereby avoiding the all-to-common reality that publications never reached those who needed them instead piling-up in a back-office room.

[37] Vietnamese would tell me they have an entrenched cultural trait that says Viet Nam is different. For example, rather than just accepting a practice common elsewhere they always needed to test it themselves (e.g., the use of Oxytocin a hormone that controls key aspects of the reproductive system, including childbirth and lactation).

in many developing countries. To tackle these, we distributed protocols for safe birth (i.e. the 'national standards') in our seven rural provinces.[38] Follow-up training to medical staff was then given. We tried to ensure the equipment provided (medical, audio-visual) was actually used and, if so, was regularly serviced by a trained technician who had access to spare parts.[39] Management information systems were introduced, and staff trained on how to maintain them (although we were never sure that the clinics had sufficient clients to justify their existence)[40] We also endeavoured to instil the message that once UNFPA funded a building or financed a training programme, that was not the end of the project, but rather, the beginning. And we tried to focus on the 'target audiences', the remote, the poor and the minorities, and not just the administrators and service providers.

Impacting on these initiatives were the unique factors of a one-party state. The key government counterparts kept a very tight rein on the role of aid agencies. Commendable was the insistence that all UN funding be spent in the country and not consumed by outsiders. But this meant any questioning of operations, calls for changes and proposed diverting of funds were often difficult. The recipient ministries under the authority of MPI zealously guarded their projects and their personnel. Not surprisingly, with each succeeding country programme, little changed. The same objectives with the

---

[38]Though we were continually told that the biggest problem commune health centres faced was implementing the national standards.

[39]Purchasing equipment was a very large component of our country programme (as it was in many countries and remains so). It was an easy deliverable, recipients valued it and money was spent. But its utility often needed questioning. In our case, did it reach the commune health clinic or was it siphoned off at the district? Was the new equipment being used or sitting on the floor, still unopened in its original packaging? Perhaps the assembly instructions were in English, power was intermittent, or a key part was missing. Also routinely noticed was the absence of our UNFPA funded posters or booklets (e.g., those spelling out the correct guidelines and procedures for RH care). On occasions we did find some, they could be bundled together, and piled in a corner of a room, collecting dust. I was often reminded of the office in Beijing with its spare room containing piles of old publications never distributed.

[40]Time and again when our team would visit a clinic, be in the morning or afternoon, there were never any clients or very few of them. A reason was always given but you began to doubt the clinic's utility especially when compared to the crowds attending the district or regional hospital, leading to patient overload, or for those who could afford it, the private clinics such as those funded by Marie Stopes Viet Nam.

same projects with the same counterparts delivering the same training using the same equipment year after year.[41]/[42] It was time for a change.

As Viet Nam moved towards middle-income status it became more and more important for the UN to respond strategically to the policy priorities of the country. There was a realisation that the system was not operating as effectively as it could, and that we risked becoming irrelevant. From this genesis was born the One UN movement, an undertaking that increasingly engaged all of us.

In September 2005 two of my colleagues, Jordan Ryan, the UNDP Representative and UN Resident Coordinator, and Jesper Morch, the UNICEF Representative, circulated a discussion paper titled "United Nations Reform: A Country Perspective".[43] Their paper was timed to coincide with the 2005 World Summit in New York where the future of UN aid was a key item on the agenda. It was also in response to calls by agency heads to harmonise services such as the procurement of equipment, translation charges, mileage allowances, driver's uniforms, and payments for photocopy paper. But Jordan and Jesper went further than these so-called 'easy wins'. They strongly critiqued the country operations of the UN system, arguing that its presence in Viet Nam was vulnerable to charges of loss of focus, incompetence, and irrelevance. They pointed to the hypocrisy whereby the UN urged donors to reform, while its own agencies, funds and programmes persisted with their age-old habits of poor coordination and loss of substance. They described a situation where the UN concentrated all its technical expertise in HQ and regional centres, while hollowing out its country

---

[41] Our work with ethnic groups provided a clear illustration of this repetitive trap. Given their high mortality rates, the idea was conceived that midwives needed to be trained to provide emergency obstetric care to these groups. Programme after programme continued the project. Justification was found, brochures were printed, and donors funded. It was much lauded. But when it was looked at from an analytical perspective, none of the midwives trained were delivering babies because they only had an 8th grade education and were not given permission by the Ministry of Health to deliver Oxytocin needed to stop bleeding. They never saved any lives. In fact, by not referring women to clinics with life-saving facilities, instead keeping them at home, they threatened their lives. It was only a rigorous evaluation that persuaded the government to rework this project. Revealed again was the importance, not only of evaluation, but of the bind that national staff find themselves in when pressured by government or are pre-occupied with managing projects and or are unable, or unwilling, to engage in policy leadership.

[42] No project should ever start without a substantive evaluation included. Such was revealed when the money that went to creating "youth friendly corners" at commune health centres was found to be significantly wasted owing to under-utilisation. Not surprising when you consider that to get to a 'corner' a youth had to walk through the clinic in view of everyone. "They feel embarrassed especially when the staff know their parents," commune health worker.

[43] Had I not been on home leave at the time, I would certainly have been involved in the drafting and added my name to the paper.

offices that were increasingly staffed by JPO's and volunteers.[44] The lack of coordination, they concluded (and I along with them), saw the agencies increasingly marginalised, and outdone by other, better resourced, multilateral organisations more equipped to promote human rights and democratic governance.[45]

Underpinning their case was the reality there were 28 major bilateral donors active in Viet Nam in 2005, and 16 separate UN agencies housed in ten different locations in Ha Noi (plus the World Bank, the Asian Development Bank and an estimated 500 NGO's). Although Overseas Development Assistance (ODA) accounted for a third of the Vietnamese budget at the time,[46] the UN agencies accounted for only 2% of this (with UNFPA's share only 0.4%). More telling was that each agency was located in their own offices, with separate representatives, and separate staff, budgets, structures, counterparts, programmes, objectives, and time frames. In their paper Jordan and Jesper illustrated the lack of coordination through the example of employing security guards:

> In Viet Nam, UNDP and UNICEF share a main gate, but each agency hires its own security guard. Visitors to the UN office in Viet Nam are still greeted by two individuals, one representing UNDP and one UNICEF. If the agencies are unable to work out how to rotate security guards, they are unlikely to reach agreement on the appropriate division of labour in delivering a substantive development programme on the ground.

Given the duplication it was inevitable there was competition for funding and for policy influence between agencies, and between agencies and other donors.[47] This led to 'mission creep', the search for more projects deemed necessary to finance an agency's continued presence in-country.[48] For example, UNFPA, UNESCO, WHO, UNAIDS, UNICEF, IOM and

---

[44]A 'reality' not unlike what I discovered at HQ'and sought to change through the "Field Needs Assessment Project", See Chap. 9.

[45]In the words of the Swedish Ambassador, "For the Europeans, the question is do they put their money into the EC or the UN. In future, we will go through the EC." Heads of Agency Retreat, 23 January 2006.

[46]Vice Minister Dat, MPI, briefing a delegation of the European Commission to Vietnam, 1 September 2004. Viet Nam was the biggest recipient of ODA per capita in the world at that time.

[47]One of our major strategies was the 'capacity building' (try as we might it was always difficult to escape the language of UN assistance.) of government partners at national, provincial, district and commune levels, and through this ensure that the Vietnamese government had ownership over its aid. This was not always easy because of the siloed structure of the Vietnamese ministries and because it was very difficult to obtain an organisational chart for each of our local partners.

[48]Only four UN agencies were self-financing—UNDP, UNICEF, UNFPA and WHO. The remainder had to raise money in-country to maintain their presence. Thus, the competition for scarce donor funds.

UNDP were all administering similar projects, with different ministries, under the euphemism that they were 'cross-cutting'. Areas covered included migration, adolescents, safe motherhood and new-born health, gender, school curriculums and data collection.[49] To the increasing irritation of government, the UN was simply taking on too many jobs and continuously multiplying its functions, a classic UN response to external challenges.

The concept of there being One UN was a confronting message which, when initially circulated at HQs, was not well received. But New York's negative response was only the first of many challenges our country team had to face. What followed was a long and, at times, tortuous navigation through uncertain waters. Our path to reform took its toll particularly among the senior UN leaders in Viet Nam. In common with most proposed transitions, from business as usual to something different, there were those that supported, those who simply went along and those who either openly or subversively opposed. Significant though was that the government,[50] and the donors,[51] wanted change. This was made apparent in my very first meeting with the Deputy Director, Foreign Economic Relations Department, MPI (my counterpart). In November 2004 he bemoaned the institutional arrangements whereby each agency had different requirements. "It's not fair," he declared, "each agency having different planning cycles. It's very difficult. What we want is one joint programme, not the occasional joint programming by multiple agencies we have at present."[52] Equally significant, from my perspective, was that UNFPA's regional and global directors agreed that

---

[49]Compounding the situation was that our counterparts could not always understand the terminology used. For example,'gender sensitive' was a commonly used developmental term which constantly required clarification.

[50]We did not need to look far to see that the government was totally committed to an aid effectiveness agenda. This was evident in the 2005 Ha Noi Core Statement on Aid Effectiveness, a Vietnamese version of the OECD Paris Declaration on Aid Effectiveness. In it the Government states its determination to reduce excessive administration of aid and cut unnecessary government costs. It proposed to do this through increased government ownership of development policies, strengthened donor alignment, improved in-country systems, stronger institutional capacity, and the simplification of development procedures and accountability. Despite the fact that the UN system accounted for so little ODA, it was the government's view that the UN was a primary source of aid ineffectiveness, especially, when dealing with 11 separate agencies. But they were more than willing to support our reform efforts given the long relationship (and the fact that we maintained a country presence when most bilateral agencies stayed away post the American War).

[51]By February 2006, 11 bilateral donors in Viet Nam were said to be 'inspired' by our initiative (Notes from a 'One UN' meeting, MPI, 22 February 2006). "You have no choice" said the DFID representative, "you either make the most of this process or you won't have any more funding. You have to be bold and provide strategic leadership, not more and more projects" (Notes, January 2008).

[52]He was also being pressured by the World Bank. As it became more of a grant-making institution, the Bank was beginning to encroach on the domain once 'naturally' occupied by the UN. For example, the Bank was supporting the VCFPC's Behaviour Change Communication (BCC) Strategy, an area traditionally supported by UNFPA. Neither the Bank nor VCPFC sought any consultation with UNFPA on the potential overlap in our 7 provinces each of which had a BCC Strategy. Being

the UN's field operations required change, and radical change at that. They argued that the system needed to commit to coordination, adopt a clear system-wide focus, and pool resources and energies to fulfil the shared agenda of the UN Charter and the MDGs. In brief, move beyond the rhetoric and actually achieve operational unity. Otherwise, face increasing irrelevance.

Accordingly, a complete reform in Viet Nam was proposed. Underpinned by Jordan and Jesper's call for change, a detailed "Roadmap" was prepared in January 2006 by the representatives of the ExCom agencies, UNDP, UNICEF and UNFPA.[53] Placing our initiative within the larger context of the Paris Declaration on Aid Effectiveness and its Viet Nam adaption, the Ha Noi Core Statement of Aid Effectiveness, we spelt out five unifying pillars

- One leader, to ensure accountability and transparency
- One plan, to ensure that we were working together
- One budget and one fund, to ensure unification
- One Set of Management Practices (finance, software, personnel) and
- One House.

Initially, our One UN effort was confined to just the three excom agencies. The specialised agencies did not immediately join. To accommodate their differing governance structures, and programmes, a two-track system was agreed to, whereby they could join when they were ready.[54] Along with donors and government ministries (MPI, MOF, MOFA and OofG) a specially created Tripartite National Task Force (TNTF) was then formed to discuss steps and risks.[55] Radical reforms were mooted. Quick wins were called for. The first move came in May 2006 when the TNTF proposal titled "Agreed Principles, Objectives, and Instruments to Achieve One United Nations in Vietnam" was approved by the Prime Minister. The next came in mid-2006 when UNAIDS, UNIFEM, and UNV joined the original three. Later, in 2007, the eight specialised agencies (FAO, IFAD, ILO, UNESCO, UNIDO, UNCTAD, UNODC, and WHO) chose to participate, and in June 2008 all fourteen participating agencies approved a new One Plan/One

---

able to make much bigger donations and grants meant the Bank had more policy leverage and influence.

[53]So-called because they were members of the UN Development Group Executive Committee.

[54]Gaining approval from their respective headquarters proved not to be automatic. Some were concerned about a loss of profile valuing the special relationships built up with counterpart ministries, and others were fearful of what was viewed as a UNDP push for ascendency.

[55]The donors, particularly the Dutch, French, Norwegians and British, were frustrated at the slow pace of reforms. Supporting them were Australia, Canada, Ireland, Japan, Luxembourg, New Zealand, and Singapore.

Budget, a combination of all their planning documents.[56] Whilst not perfect, it was, in the words of one representative, the best we could do.

The sense that Viet Nam was creating history really came with the development of the One Plan and One Budget, which were formulated by teams consisting of the office of the Resident Coordinator, staff from the agencies, and our government counterparts. Chaired by the deputy director, MPI, they combined each agencies' country programmes, and their accompanying budgets, into a common plan. Critical overall was the intent to make the coordination and delivery of aid programmes much easier by reducing programme overlap and waste.[57] Important from a UNFPA perspective was that it was driven by the goals and core values set out by the ICPD.

The signs that we were moving at a pace that was uncomfortable for New York, came via a telephone conference in April 2006. "Things seem to be moving a bit too quickly", a representative of the UN Development Group (UNDG) told us.[58] "The principles have said 'do not go too far'". By August

---

[56]While the specialised agencies are linked to the United Nations through individual agreements with ECOSOC, "...the intergovernmental bodies charged with oversight and coordination of the economic and social work of the UN system, in particular ECOSOC, perform poorly. It could scarcely be otherwise given the extraordinary mishmash of organisations governments have created." Evidence that the UN Secretary-General cannot give directions to the heads of these agencies, who are legally answerable only to their own plenary bodies. Ingram op cit p. 10. The new plan was known as One Plan II to distinguish it from the original One Plan I which remained unique to the Excoms being based on the CPAPs. That financial distinction between I and II was later a source of much friction. The SAs could not access OPI.

[57]The lack of system-wide coherence was an issue taken up by UN Secretary-General Kofi Annan as early as July 1997. Then, at the 2005 World Summit Assembly, he called for reinforcement of management and the coordination of UN operational activities. It was reasoned that this was necessary for the UN to contribute more effectively to its objectives, primarily, the MDGs. In February 2006, the Secretary-General announced the creation of a high-level panel of experts charged with exploring the UN system and how it could work more coherently and effectively. In response, the Vietnamese Deputy Prime Minister wrote to the Secretary General asking that Viet Nam be designated a pilot country to implement the recommendations of the HLP report. Several months later in November, the 'Delivering as One' report was delivered and a programme in the same name was launched in 8 pilot countries: Albania, Cape Verde, Mozambique, Pakistan, Rwanda, Tanzania, Uruguay, and Viet Nam. Recommended was that "the UN accelerate and deepen reforms to establish unified UN country teams-with one leader, one programme, and one budgetary framework and, where appropriate, one office." While this created a clear timeline for a reform process it was top down. Papers emanating from New York were seen as just paper exercises. UN reform, as I knew it, did not originate as a result of the 2005 World Summit. Inertia, rules, lack of specificity, divisions among different agencies, and special interests meant continued procrastination. In Viet Nam it was the efforts of the UN Team, the donors, and the government that kick started the global effort. We deliberately called it 'One UN' so there would be no equivocation of what we intended. The more opportunistic but less rigorous 'Delivering as One' could mean whatever you wanted it to.

[58]The UNDG is one of the three pillars of the UN system's Chief Executives Board (CEB), which furthers coordination and cooperation on a wide range of substantive and management issues. The CEB brings the executive heads of UN organizations together on a regular basis under the chairmanship of the Secretary-General.

our RC was telling us there was no clear signal coming from agency heads. "They are running hot and cold, calling for more time and leaving it up to us to determine the content of our reforms. Don't expect guidance." Following the visit to Ha Noi of the UNDG Chair in November, the message was clearer. "Viet Nam may be at the forefront of something very important, and far ahead of New York, but move cautiously. Reform is challenging, complicated, tricky." The brakes were being applied. More importantly, divisions had begun to emerge in Viet Nam.

Chief among these were the range of positions adopted by the specialised agencies. Some were keenly supportive, others were not. Some said they would only join if there were additional funds. Meanwhile, they would await guidance from their headquarters. And, in one case, when it came to the concerned Director General he was quoted as saying he was committed but didn't know how much. In another case, the local representative was reprimanded for diluting their name brand under cover of "One UN". In yet another, they rejected signposting the UN as the UNCT insisting it read UN Agencies. There were also suspicions that this was primarily a UNDP driven exercise leading to one agency head declaring that the "One Leader and One Plan was not the best approach". Then there were those who saw the donors as having too much say. Finally, a number of the smaller agencies insisted on equating their contribution to the One Plan to not just the output coming from their limited country presence but to the periodic inputs they also received from their regional offices and headquarters. Such inflation was roundly rejected by a determination that what mattered was in-country capacity and not a twice-yearly visit by a Bangkok adviser. These ad hoc claims not only demonstrated an absence of clear direction from varying headquarters but an initiative that was being individually driven. Alongside the committed core of government, donor, and agency representatives seeking a system wide reform there were those who saw no further than advancing the interests of their agency, gaining leverage far beyond what was historically the case.[59]

Throughout the often convoluted and time-consuming forward movement a number of other persistent challenges presented themselves. Most were overcome but a number were intractable, and I suspect continue to stymie UN reform to this day. Chief among these was that there were simply to many

---

[59]MPI foresaw this declaring at one stage they did not want 15 viewpoints on everything but non-interference in each other's programme was, and remains, the accepted UN practice.

agencies with very small programmes.[60] To give all their goals equal weighting without prioritisation not only minimised impact but diluted effort. Called for was a powerful leader who had the authority to take on an agency representative when they claimed ground that was clearly not theirs. While we foresaw this in Viet Nam, agreeing to a "One Leader Memorandum of Understanding," which gave the RC final decision-making power on the allocation of funds, the RC could still not instruct agencies to only work in certain programme areas. Lacking this authority, plus a disinclination to face down the autonomy of the specialised agencies, the RC's position was well-nigh impossible.[61] Extraordinary as it seemed at the time, I suspect our Viet Nam experience was the same for the remaining pilot reform countries if not the 140 countries where the UN and its agencies had a presence. Such was the vacuum in which we were charting our course, each country was deciding its own blueprint.[62]

Budgets typified the RC's powerlessness. Take UNFPA's, for example. It was based on the amount of resources coming from headquarters, plus what we believed could be realistically raised from donors and then successfully disbursed (i.e. "resource based" budgeting). Other agencies, however, based their budgets on the amount of funds they felt were needed to deliver their programmes ("needs based") irrespective of whether they could raise them or not. They included everything, including extra staff, in the hope the funds could be found. The data tells the story. In 2007 the 16 UN agencies disbursed US$62 million. The five-year total budget for One Plan was US$419 million, an annual disbursement requirement of nearly US$84 million, US$22 million more. And, of this amount, UNFPA, using a resource-based allocation, requested a 16% increase, WHO a 70% increase, and the much smaller UNIDO with only 3 staff, a 560% increase. Had UNIDO ever delivered such a big programme? No, Government never saw

---

[60]As is the case with UNFPA Country Programmes. Too many projects means limited monitoring, superficial evaluation and too much administration.

[61]Agencies were also suspicious of the connection between the RC and UNDP. We established a "firewall" between the RC and UNDP to ensure an impartial UNCT leader. To resolve this dilemma globally, a decision from the SG's office would later be required. The RC can now be recruited from anywhere in the system.

[62]A reality that was confirmed following a visit to New York by our RC in early 2007 (along with representatives from the other pilot countries). He returned telling us that at HQs reform was still just a vision, there was no one generic approach, and that what was being said now was very different to what was said earlier. In summary, he said, not knowing who was following who, it was 'chaotic and defensive'.

the need. Could they in the future? Very doubtful.[63] This was a grab for money, project driven rather than integrated programming, activity-based not results-based. The fact that UNIFEM, IFAD, HABITAT, and UNEP only opened up offices in Ha Noi after the One Plan Fund was announced further illustrates the point. We were all supposedly about policy dialogue not infrastructure spending.

Programme coordination illustrated this dichotomy very clearly. Eleven Programme Coordination Groups (PCG's) were formed in May 2008. These were the technical working groups where the UNCT would work together to jointly implement the 11 key areas of the OP. Included were (1) Social and Development Policies, (2) Trade, Employment and Enterprise Development, (3) HIV, (4) Gender, (5) Health and Reproductive Rights, (6) Protection, (7) Education, (8) Sustainable Development, (9) Governance, (10) Natural Disasters and Emergencies, (11) Communicable Diseases, Zoonoses and other Animal Diseases. Through annual work plans the aim was to jointly analyse and reduce overlaps. Members were accountable to both their agency and to the PCG. But, not surprisingly, with total UN assistance measuring only 2% of aid to Viet Nam, it was not possible to deliver on every area that each of the 15 agencies prioritised. The deliberations of the respective groups began, not unreasonably, with the agency most 'prominent' in the area assuming the chairing. For agencies with multiple themes, they sought to lead more than one PCG. As it transpired, lacking prioritisation between the eleven PCGs, and in the absence of strong leadership, everything was placed on the table. Everyone sought to accommodate everyone, even those who could not re-programme their resources owing to commitments already signed. Letting go of your 'shopping list', achievable or otherwise, funded or not, proved an enormous challenge. Staff not only inflated their agency's earlier programmes, but also continually elevated its future needs in anticipation that the extra funds coming from donors would pay for more staff. The result was a One Plan of 320 outputs (later repackaged to 152) and 35 outcome indicators. It was simply about wanting more money without changing anything. This meant the One Fund was never allocated according to an objective prioritisation (i.e., our anticipated new method of delivering results based on a holistic approach of what the UN could actually deliver to the country's social and economic development).[64] In the absence of reality,

---

[63] Even UNFPA had trouble disbursing its funds. In March 2007 US$129 million was unspent globally and had to be returned to donors. This amount was out of an annual budget of US$600 million.

[64] Regrettably, reaching consensus is still problematic today. Evidence clashes over ownership of the water, sanitation, and hygiene (WASH) programme between WFP and UNICEF.

agencies continued to spend their own funds using their own procurement rules and regulations, a reversion to 'business as usual.'[65]/[66]

These barriers to progress led to a questioning of the UN's capacity to deliver a reform agenda. Repeatedly, at team retreats, there was debate about the purpose of the assistance being provided. Posed were questions about the UN's strategic position. If we were not a donor, were we an advocate and, if so, for what? Human rights, norms and standards or simply stated, better service to government and to people? And, if the latter, which people? It was said to be the poor but was it again that 'symbiotic relationship between government elites, UN elites and NGO elites'? In turn, this led to questioning how much would really change. Was our One UN just a paper exercise? "Were the shoes pinching or were we still safe in our comfort zones?" Were we, after all, just a self-satisfied group of aging representatives salving our consciences for what we should have done? Over-promising and under-delivering. Even though we never quite answered these questions, we committed to carrying on, to 'just do it'.

Over the three years of my involvement with this pioneering exercise there was, not surprisingly, much adaption as we were learning by doing. From its inception in early 2006 until my departure in early 2009, we were besieged by the amount of time and resources it took. Under One Plan there was a steering committee and a management allocation committee. Then there were the sub-sets requiring long and, at times, tedious discussion and resolution (an affliction endemic to the UN). Under Management Practices there was not only a plan to be resolved but also agreement on harmonising common services, cash transfers, cost norms, project management guidelines and communication strategies. And, because implementation of the entire initiative required a significant change in behaviour, surveys of staff attitudes towards change were required as were team building exercises once capacities were assessed and constraints identified. Finally, the success of the transformation required confirmation from our partners in the government and outside (e.g., donors, NGO's, community organisations and the business sector) that

---

[65]The allocation process was not helped by a deliberate decision of MPI's. The ministry insisted on grouping together, into one, each of the "Country Programme Action Plans" (CPAPs) of all the participating agencies. They had already been agreed to, the government maintained, with all of the counterpart ministries expecting their negotiated programme of assistance. Consequently, there was no clean slate.

[66]Later a formula was agreed to whereby previous yearly fund allocations, 2001–2005, were used as a guide to how much could be claimed but a number of agencies refused to comply and insisted their grossly inflated programmes were achievable. For example, one agency insisted on ramping up its programme from US$1 million to US$12 million. It was a blatant grab for money.

the change undertaken was substantive and not just cosmetic. Donors particularly needed to be kept informed of progress. Increased funding was a key goal.

There was also much disagreement about an assortment of practical issues which delayed implementation. For a year and a half, agencies debated membership of the various committees and the necessary procedural details. Many wanted their counterparts from the line ministries included and not just the members of the "Government Aid Coordinating Agencies" (OofG, MOF, MOFA and MPI). Restrictions were also placed on the harmonisation of business practices, for example, cash transfers by some agency headquarters. All of us had to be mandated from our headquarters to experiment and most were authorised to go ahead. For reluctant participants, however, constant referrals were made, required or not. Even when it came to signing key documents many agencies questioned what signing signified. They were concerned that signing meant full compliance.[67]

Another of the persistent challenges was language. We struggled with the standard rhetoric typical of the UN workplace. Hours were spent debating what an 'outcome' meant. If that was a challenge for the English speakers, the Vietnamese word for output (e.g. printing a book) and outcome (reading it) was the same. Even more problematic for the Vietnamese were terms common in UN speak—cost norms, systemic issues, quality assurance, gender sensitive, capacity building, national execution, evidence based, value added, transaction costs, operational support, and opportunity cost. Agreeing on these resulted in endless discussions, often inconclusive. As the number of meetings intensified pages of definitions plus acronyms were required. Given these complexities, and the time taken with little to show, tensions became fraught. As a result, many agency heads delegated responsibilities to over-burdened national staff who in turn passed it on to JPOs, UNVs and interns.[68] Lacking detailed knowledge of programme and administrative procedures they were often "out of their depth" and lacked authority to make decisions.

The final pillar of our reform initiative proved to be the least challenging. It was the building of *One UN House*. By the end of 2007 we aimed to have a single location instead of multiple offices across Ha Noi. Being all in the same building, the goal was to bring down barriers, thereby fostering a sense of common 'identity'. We saw staff sitting together according to function

---

[67]Government was also irritated with the amount of time being taken. When it came to business practices, they proposed we adopt their administrative and financial procedures. Because this was contrary to standard UN regulations it was never accepted.

[68]Because of the increased workload, I was able to temporarily hire additional staff as well as allocate two existing staff members to work on the exercise.

rather than agency. Facilitating their coherence would be agreement on a set of "Harmonised Project/Programme Management Guidelines (HPPMG)", whereby business procedures would be aligned, technical support pooled, and common services simplified. We wanted to save money by standardising IT and the maintenance of office equipment. Adding to the vision, the One House was to be a carbon neutral building, a 'green house'.

The relevant committee overseeing the project was chaired by a representative of the Ministry of Foreign Affairs (MFA). From the start the initiative received almost unanimous support. Not surprising, really. Donors like bricks and mortar just as UNFPA likes equipment and contraceptives. Unlike changing behaviour, hardware is visible and an easy spend. Initially, One House was not without its challenges. A number of agencies did not want to contribute financially, because they enjoyed rent-free premises or paid below market rates. Others inflated the number of staff they had leading to a reprimand aired at a heads of agency meeting that the aim of our reform was not to create a bigger UN but a smaller one. By the time of my departure donors had contributed US$5 million of the US$7 million required with the government agreeing to make up the difference. The proposed Green One UN House was to be a concrete manifestation of our reform efforts.[69]/[70]

When I left Viet Nam the general feeling was that UN reform had a better chance of success than comparable efforts in other countries. There was strong government support, equally strong donor support, and a strong

---

[69]The building was inaugurated in May 2015 by then UN Secretary-General, Ban Ki-moon and Viet Nam's Deputy Prime Minister and Minister of Foreign Affairs. Among the very first globally to realise such an ambition, with most resident UN agencies having decided to move in, most staff were located according to function.

[70]Five years later, in 2020, agency staff informed me that colocation had increased coordination and collaboration. But, they said, it depended on the availability of funding and the personality of the agency head. "In the 6 years I've served in Viet Nam", one colleague told me, "the One UN approach ebbed and flowed. When representatives were willing to cooperate and pay for their share, aspects flourished." Others declared that some heads of agencies saw One-UN as stepping on their territory and "...slammed on the brakes in the UNCT". Another told me that as Viet Nam moved into "lower middle-income country" status funding came largely through agencies and not country donors (the Dutch left in 2012). This meant that, in their opinion, agencies were less keen to share their resources. An 'absurd example' given was that every agency still bought "...their own fancy cars with sharing of vehicles not something that was routinely done". And you also had situations "...where you could not even find money for a simple brownbag lunch. Staff paid those things out of their own pocket". Conclusion? As in other transformative UN initiatives, agency take-up was not organisationally driven but dependent on personalities.

core of UN staff committed to the principles of One UN.[71] An Irish mission in late 2008 summed it up as follows

> There is no comparison between 2005 when you started and now. It may not be ideal, but the genie is out of the bottle and you will never return to the way it was done. UN headquarters may not have changed but your pilot has.

Despite this affirmation, a mood of pessimism pervaded the UNCT. We had aimed to reform a self-satisfied but under-performing system, but after enormous time and effort we seemed to have gone round in a full circle. No longer were we talking greater efficiencies, better data, better analysis, fewer key strategic results, but just endless joint programming with endless guidelines. 'Enhanced coherence' was now the goal rather than complete financial and programme integration. When staff returned to their offices, agency overload took precedence. The silos had not seen a change of mindset. By giving every agency equal weight, the UN family was not so loving as we thought. Perhaps a new team could move beyond our lowest common denominator.[72]

For myself leaving Viet Nam was the end of my UN career or so I imagined. Having joined in the seventies UN rules now dictated retirement. Everyone came to the airport. A reception room was booked, and we sat around reminiscing about the wonderful times we had had. A special place and a special time. Then we were on the plane heading off to our next posting, only this time it was home.

---

[71]Strong central government providing public goods, like health care, is a feature of modern Viet Nam. This explains, in part, the effective way the country dealt with the COVIC-19 pandemic. As of April 2020, not a single death had been recorded even though a border is shared with China although by August of the same year, such was the challenge of the virus, that an outbreak in Da Nang had led to new infections.

[72]At the last HOA meeting I attended in December 2008 the RC reported that the mood in New York was one of "…malaise, a lack of interest, of waiting out the pilot phase in the field so they could get back to their own agendas." This mirrored my own observation when I visited HQs in late October. Everybody was frantically busy, but it had little or no bearing with what we were frantically busy with in Viet Nam.

11

Life After Death: Rwanda

"The past is not dead. In fact, it's not even past." William Faulkner

Retirement.[1] In 2009 I returned to my hometown of Melbourne after an absence of forty years. Very lost. I moped around. "What to do?" Monday morning would come and I wanted to head off to work just as I had over thirty years of assignments. But here in Melbourne there was no office, no local contacts, no agenda. There were no old mates to talk to. My colleagues were all overseas, pursuing their UN careers or, like me, retired. As I scrambled for something to do, I couldn't help looking up, longingly, as aeroplanes flew overhead. The black dog was on me. The family suffered too. "Get over it!" But it was hard. Had I learnt anything about transition strategies since my return from Texas 45 years earlier? At night I dreamt, only to force myself awake to record a message I had clearly heard. "Engage the world. Mental imprisonment is gone forever." Then it happened. I received a call asking if I was interested in a temporary position as officer-in-charge of the Rwanda UNFPA Office. Hallelujah! I was not forgotten. I leapt at the idea, although I appreciated that heading off to a relatively unknown country in the centre of Africa was not something everybody would welcome. For me, however, it felt normal. Afterall, it was what I had always done throughout my career.

---

[1]The personnel rules of the UN applicable to me at that time required staff members who joined before 1 January 1990 to retire at 60 years and those that joined thereafter at 62. For those joining now it is 65.

© The Author(s), under exclusive license to Springer Nature Switzerland AG 2021
I. Howie, *Reflections on a United Nations' Career*, Springer Biographies, https://doi.org/10.1007/978-3-030-77063-1_11

Nonetheless preparing for a new country assignment still brought with it waves of anxiety. Travelling alone, leaving the family behind, arriving at an unknown destination and navigating the first weeks in a foreign land, would present many challenges.

I arrived in Rwanda in mid-December 2009. Even though I had served in Africa, and undertaken many missions there, I had never visited Rwanda. Sure, I knew where the country was and that it was a troubled nation with a history of genocide—something to do with Hutus and Tutsis. But who were these groups, and how did they interact? I scarcely knew.

I arrived, genuinely feeling I was in the middle of the continent, but puzzled by the climate knowing I was on the equator. Where was the humidity? The answer soon became apparent. Rwanda is a high-altitude country of rivers, a 'thousand' hills and, surprisingly, eucalyptus trees. As I flew into the capital, I saw below me snaking rivers, dirt roads lined by orderly rows of wooden houses, an abundance of lakes, few trees and intense cultivation: a patchwork of brown hues.

My first challenge came after I had cleared immigration at the airport and stood waiting to collect my luggage. I was on the defensive when a young man came up to me and asked, somewhat furtively or so it seemed to me, if I had any plastic bags. Being new, and apprehensive, I asked myself why I was being approached by this unknown person even before I had stepped out of the terminal. No doubt he had had this reaction before because he then patiently explained to me that plastic bags were not allowed in the country. "Could I please deposit mine in the bin placed there for that purpose," he asked. I did as I was told. So began my first lesson into modern Rwanda.

Once outside the terminal I nervously scanned the waiting crowd. Ah, there was the UNFPA name sign being held up. Whew! "Welcome, sir." "No, please call me Ian," I replied. He looked startled. Such informality was not what he expected from the representative. Nor did he expect me to sit in the front seat eager to chat. Clearly, there was an established pattern of behaviour where the protocol set was to fly the flag and have the door opened for you. To build trust I would need to understand the roots of this. As I was driven to my hotel I saw what seemed to be a reserved city when compared with other African capitals. Either by disposition or poverty, or history, people were walking quietly. They were not boisterous. There were no motorbikes or bicycles, few cars and most people either paid to ride in a minivan or walked. And the streets were spotlessly clean. Even the roadside dust was swept into piles, scooped up and disposed of. The numbers of young men standing around or walking along the road suggested unemployment was a challenge.

I asked myself how it was possible that Kigali was not noisy, congested and dirty like most other cities in developing countries. The UN driver gave me the answer. On the last Saturday of every month, he said, the entire population from the President down were required to join their local community in cleaning up the neighbourhood and collaborating on important public works. This practice, called *Umuganda,* causes the country to come to a complete halt. No traffic, no pedestrians, just people cleaning up.[2] But who was this president able to enforce such behaviour? Was he a charismatic demagogue? A military dictator, hiding behind a screen of populism? Or was he the typical African 'big man', in power for decades, ruling via his tribal cronies and corruption? My first impressions suggested that after the horrors of the genocide in 1994, the country seemed to have picked itself up, albeit under the dictates of a very tough leader. Given my earlier African experience of an entrenched elite enriching itself, already hinted was a very different type of ruler.

The hotel where I spent the first week was across the road from the UN building. On day one I went to the office, keen to meet the staff. They were astonished I had come at all after such a long flight. Everyone was friendly but I sensed wariness, in part explained by the horrific ethnic history of the country and, in part, by what I discovered the staff had experienced in the preceding few years. Because I had received no prior briefing—nothing unusual there—I only knew there was a representative vacancy needing to be filled. Experience had taught me that when you're parachuted into an office and greeted cautiously, there was a history that needed to be understood and massaged into a more positive outlook. Later, I came to learn that following the resignation of two of the three senior staff members, and the evaporation of any sense of team spirit, the staff had written to the regional office prompting it to move the representative to another country. Rightly or wrongly, she was viewed as combative, elitist, and a perfectionist to the point of dysfunction. Following her relocation, the office continued to deal with routine programme delivery under another temporary representative, but it was now expected of me to build the team into a dynamic unit.

In common with other country postings, my first few days required me to attend the mandatory security briefing from the UN security officer. I was informed that the situation in Kigali was thought of as safe, and comparable to those of the better run African capitals. However, there had been

---

[2]Read more about *Umuganda* on the Rwanda Governance Board website: http://www.rgb.rw/index.php?id=37.

six random grenade attacks since 2008, and I was advised not to frequent public places, to avoid movement after 6 p.m. and to be alert to my surroundings. While everything seemed quiet, the security officer advised me that you never knew what was bubbling under the surface. A hand grenade thrown at a bus station soon after I arrived highlighted his concerns. What didn't help was that all the security warnings coming from the UN were either written or spoken in French. When I pointed out that this wasn't conducive to calming the anxieties of the English-speaking staff, myself included, and that the country had formally changed the medium of education from French to English in 2008, I was viewed as being demanding. Fortunately, although only after repeated interventions, it was seen that understanding the security announcements could be critical in a crisis. This required them to be made in French and English.

After a week, I left the familiarity of a hotel and moved to an empty house, located in a very quiet but affluent suburb. I had taken up the very kind offer of my deputy to stay in his house while he went on leave. This took the pressure off having to find somewhere to live, especially when rents were high. Sitting alone in that house, the coming months stretching before me seemed a very long time. I thought of home and had moments wondering how I would cope with the loneliness. But I also thought of the challenges Rwanda faced, and asked myself what I knew of the life Rwandans had lived and were now living? I concluded that it was up to me to do some small thing in the months ahead for both the Rwandans and myself.

As these snapshots of my first days in the country suggested, one could not visit Rwanda let alone live there without confronting one of the most horrific events of the last century. How did an estimated 300,000 people of the largest ethnic group set about exterminating 800,000 of another when both spoke the same language, observed the same customs and worshipped the same God, and do so at a rate three times faster than that of the Holocaust?[3] And how did a small landlocked country of 10 million people, without any natural resources, manage to rehabilitate itself from a situation of total destruction, to an elevated status as one of Africa's success stories? I don't pretend to have anything but superficial answers but here is a pocket history of a compelling narrative.

The ethnic tensions that fuelled the genocide were ignited long before 1994. We know the first inhabitants of Rwanda were a hunter-gatherer people, ancestors of the Twa who still live in Rwanda today and constitute

---

[3]Gourevitch, P 1995, 'After the Genocide', *The New Yorker*, http://www.newyorker.com/magazine/1995/12/18/after-the-genocide.

around 0.3% of the population.[4] The Twa were followed by the farming Hutus who were moving throughout Central Africa looking for fertile land. Later came the cattle-raising Tutsis ('Tutsis' means 'owners of cattle'), perhaps coming from the north or north east. Gradually, a hierarchy and master-client relationship emerged—whether by conquest or a natural process—in which cattle raisers were seen as superior to farmers.

Under a Tutsi king the country survived, tucked away as it was in the centre of Africa. Until the 1890s it managed to avoid foreign incursions, insulating itself from colonialism and the slave trade. Despite few or no Europeans ever being there, 'Ruanda-Urundi' (now Rwanda and Burundi) was parcelled out to Germany at the Berlin Conference of 1885 and incorporated into German East Africa. In 1916 Belgium invaded. With the end of World War I, it assumed control under a League of Nations mandate. In 1945, still as one country, Ruanda-Urundi became a UN Trust Territory and Belgium was charged with guiding a transition to independence.

Throughout the colonial era, alleged ethnic differences were highlighted with the Tutsis, 15% of the population claiming authority over the vastly more numerous Hutus. Tutsi dominance was supported by Roman Catholic missionaries who ran the schools and, through generations, systematically reinforced established power structures. While Tutsi power was slightly weakened by the introduction of Belgian administrators, the Hutu majority remained second-class citizens. In a 1930s census Rwanda's population was classified as Hutu, Tutsi or Twa, based on physical characteristics and cow ownership. Identity cards were then issued.

As more Hutus became educated, their voice grew, leaders emerged and calls were made for the Hutu majority to take power, and for drastic reform before independence. For their part, the Belgians did little to further either cause. Unlike earlier, the Catholic Church was now pro-Hutu, and supported the formation of political parties.

In July 1959, the King died under mysterious circumstances. There were outbreaks of sporadic violence and suggestions of Belgian involvement. By November these had grown much larger and over a period of around two weeks, 20,000–100,000 Tutsis were killed as Hutu gangs began a murderous rampage. Tutsi retaliation followed, leading to the country being placed under military rule and Tutsis leaving as refugees. But a pro-Hutu party won the 1961 election and introduced quotas limiting the number of education

---

[4]According to the World Directory of Minorities and Indigenous Peoples, Minority Rights Group International, http://minorityrights.org/minorities/twa-2/.

places and jobs for Tutsis (who had now fallen to approximately 9% of the population).

In the early 1970s, following further crackdowns against the Tutsis and a campaign to "purify" the country, killing and violence broke out again. Amidst all this, the President was ousted by Major-General Juvénal Habyarimana who in 1975 formed a single political party with representatives "on every hill and in every cell"[5] whom Habyarimana rigidly controlled and led. While there was relative stability for a time, a fall in commodity prices and a rise in oil prices led to the economy suffering. Dissatisfaction grew. Reports of corruption and mismanagement spread. Rwandan refugees began organising themselves in Uganda.

Seeking to restore democracy the Rwandan Patriotic Front (RPF) invaded north-east Rwanda from Uganda in 1990. The RPF was formed from "The Rwandan Refugee Welfare Foundation Patriotic Front" (RPF) which itself had been formed in Uganda in 1979 and was supported by Tutsis and Hutus who opposed Habyarimana's regime. The RPF's leader, Fred Rwigyema, and subsequent leader Paul Kagame, had both played leading roles in the guerrilla war in Uganda that had overthrown President Obote in 1987. The incursion in 1990 was soon suppressed following Habyarimana's request for troops from France, Belgium and Zaire. With this foreign support the Rwandan army engaged in a rampage of reprisals against both Tutsis and any Hutus suspected of RPF collaboration. Thousands were shot or hacked to death. Others were indiscriminately arrested or herded into stadiums and police stations, where they were left without food or water. Outside pressure calling for an end to the violence led to Habyarimana agreeing to the abolition of ethnic identity cards, but nothing was implemented. Then, in 1991, as the international community continued to demand change, President Habyarimana allowed free debate on the country's future and agreed in principle to multi-party democracy. His government also set about enlarging its army as well as arming and training *interahamwe*—civilian militias. Meanwhile, in Uganda, President Museveni was keen to repatriate 250,000 Rwandan refugees. He supported the re-organising and re-equipping of the RPF. Now led by Paul Kagame, following the death of Rwigyema in the 1990 invasion, the RPF mounted countrywide guerrilla raids. In response, Habyarimana invited the RPF to a conference of other African Presidents in 1992. Months of negotiations led to the Arusha Peace Accords, which stipulated cessation of hostilities, repatriation of refugees and a transitional government—intended to see power shared between Habyarimana's regime and the

---

[5]Melvern, L 2004, CONSPIRACY TO MURDER: THE RWANDAN GENOCIDE, Verso, London, p. 10.

moderate Hutu opposition. The RPF and the Rwandan army were also to be merged, along with the deployment of a neutral international peace-keeping force. The accord, however, had little political support. Some Hutu groups in Rwanda saw it as a disastrous setback.

Tensions remained high. While the resolution establishing the United Nations Assistance Mission for Rwanda (UNAMIR) was passed in October 1993, a preoccupied United Nations reacted with no urgency. As tragedies unfolded in Somalia and Bosnia,[6] the Security Council authorised only one of the two battalions requested by the Secretary-General for the Rwandan peace force. As Canadian General Romeo Dallaire, the UNAMIR force commander, was to later write, UN officials did not consider Rwanda of strategic importance, and the operation was to be conducted 'on the cheap'.[7] Thereafter, the whole peacekeeping exercise was hampered by serious shortcomings in equipment, personnel, training, intelligence and planning. Compounding the situation was a failed coup in Burundi in October 1993 when around 350,000 fled to Rwanda. This added enormously to Rwanda's problems, increased Hutu paranoia against Tutsis and reinforced inciteful propaganda that was being broadcast by Hutu radio stations such as Radio Mille Collines.

On 6 April 1994 the plane carrying President Habyarimana home from a regional summit meeting in Arusha, along with his Burundian counterpart, President Ntaryamira, was shot down on approach to Kigali airport. While it is not known conclusively who fired the missiles, it is widely believed that Hutu extremists were behind the attack, worried that the President was going to implement the Arusha Accords. Within an hour, the Presidential Guard and Hutu militias had set up roadblocks across Kigali and began murdering Tutsis and moderate Hutus. What then occurred was a well-planned attempt at a 'final solution' to the Tutsi 'problem' perpetrated by an estimated 300,000 Hutu extremists. Following the killing of the moderate Hutu Prime Minister and her Belgian peace-keeper guards, and the withdrawal of well-trained French, Italian and Belgian troops evacuating expatriates out of the country,

---

[6]For the Americans it was the killing of 18 American servicemen in Mogadishu on 3 October 1993 and for the other members of the Security Council it was the perceived ineffectiveness of the UN Operations in Somalia (UNOSOM). A similar view surrounded the endeavours of the UN Protection Force in Croatia and Bosnia and Herzegovina (UNPROFOR) in what was an increasingly complex situation. Bosnia was happening at the same time as Rwanda but given its location in the heart of Europe was far more extensively reported than Rwanda which was at the centre of faraway Africa. Today, we see a similar underreporting with the current famines in Somalia and elsewhere on the African continent.

[7]Romeo Dallaire in a 2002 interview with Ted Koppel, 'A Good Man in Hell: General Roméo Dallaire and the Rwandan Genocide', United States Holocaust Memorial Museum, June 12 2002, https://www.ushmm.org/confront-genocide/speakers-and-events/all-speakers-and-events/a-good-man-in-hell-general-romeo-dallaire-and-the-rwanda-genocide.

the killing escalated. Thousands of Tutsis and Hutus suspected of sympathising with the RPF were butchered every day. Dismembered corpses littered the streets around Kigali. Ordinary men, women and even children joined in the carnage, caught up in a tide of blind hatred, mob mentality and fear. Nuns and priests betrayed those who tried to take refuge in churches, people were forced to murder their family and friends, and all the while radio broadcasts spread inciteful messages of hatred towards the 'Tutsi cockroaches'.[8] Dallaire requested reinforcements and a broader interpretation of the mandate.[9] Fearing a repetition of Mogadishu, the UN Secretariat ordered Dallaire not to act. By April, his military assessment was that the forces under his command could not "continue to sit on the fence in the face of all these morally legitimate demands for assistance/protection."[10] But, hiding behind legalities, the UN Security Council[11] unanimously agreed that only a token UN force remain. It was cut to 250 personnel. But the RDF in Uganda didn't wait. They launched a major offensive two days after the plane crash aimed at ending the genocide and rescuing Tutsis. Three months later, after overcoming a much larger and better equipped army, the RPF captured Kigali on July 4. With the fleeing of the Hutu government to Zaire, the RPF advanced northward and westward. Then, on July 18, they announced they had won the war and established a broad-based administration. The genocide was over. A dedicated lightly armed guerrilla force had overcome a vastly stronger army. The UN agreed and sent a force to Rwanda in late July.

Meanwhile, thousands of refugees had streamed into 'safe zones' such as Zaire. This was a crisis of its own with 2 million living in makeshift refugee camps ravaged by disease. When these camps fell under the control of the fleeing Hutu militia the killing continued. The militias built a quasi-government-in-exile and recruited troops from among the camp populations in order to mount attacks into Rwanda. By 1996 Rwanda warned that if these attacks did not cease, the consequences would be dire. What ensued was Africa's first great war, involving as many as nine national neighbours

---

[8]You can read transcripts of radio broadcasts from both the lead up to and during the genocide on the website of the Montreal Institute for Genocide and Human Rights Studies, Concordia University, https://www.concordia.ca/research/migs/resources/rwanda-radio-transcripts.html.

[9]Dallaire's so named infamous cable of 11 January 1994 to the UN spoke of military preparedness, provocation "to a civil war" and "extermination of Tutsi". Then on February 27 and March 13, he requested more troops and a broader mandate. He discusses his involvement in Rwanda in depth in his book, Dallaire, R 2004, SHAKE HANDS WITH THE DEVIL: THE FAILURE OF HUMANITY TO ACT IN RWANDA, Arrow Books, London.

[10]Dallaire discusses this April report in his book, pages 306–307 ibid.

[11]Tragically, one of the 10 elected positions on the Security Council at that time was held by a representative of the Rwandan Government who deflected away any criticism of the regime.

and costing an estimated 3–5 million deaths, mostly from disease and starvation. Since then, the situation has continued to change. Peace treaties have
been signed and alliances formed only to see proxies continue the fighting.
By the time of my arrival, Kagame had been in power for almost 10 years.
Having assumed the presidency in April 2000, in August 2003 he won an
overwhelming victory at the ballot box. Later in October, his party won an
absolute majority in the first multi-party elections. The situation in 2010
was relatively calm though, as the UN security officer had advised, you never
knew what was bubbling along under the surface.[12]

After such a history, everyone I met had a story of survival. The first came
during a field trip. It was suggested I visit Nyamata, some 40 kms from
Kigali, and there find a church which had been set aside as one of the genocide memorials. I found the church without difficulty. It was an octagonal
building. As I walked across to its entrance all was very quiet. I could see no
indication of what I was meant to look for. I poked my head in the door.
I saw only piles of old brown clothing organised into lines like spokes on
a bicycle wheel. It made little sense to me, until I was suddenly addressed
by someone running up behind me. "I am your guide," said Charles, "I am
sorry for being late, I was taking my lunch". Charles then proceeded to tell
me, in graphic detail, about the events which began on 9 April 1994. He
narrated how they happened, hour by hour. He told me how the local Tutsi
population had fled to the church, where they were surrounded by the *interahamwe*. For three days the militia shouted, beat drums and blew whistles,
while those inside went without food and water. When the army soldiers
finally arrived and their captain addressed the terrified people, many thought
their ordeal was over. They were wrong. The captain told them their day of
judgement had come. Shooting began. Over the next three weeks, 10,000 or
more people were slaughtered, mainly by machetes and clubs, in that church.
Day after day, the soldiers hacked away, only stopping for lunch and an afternoon nap, before they took up their grisly work again. To avoid the people
running away, they cut their Achilles tendons.

---

[12]For a more detailed accounts on the genocide see:

   Caplan, G 2007, 'Rwanda: Walking the Road to Genocide', in Allan Thompson (ed.), THE
MEDIA AND THE RWANDA GENOCIDE, Pluto Books, pp. 20–38.

   Dallaire, R 2004, SHAKE HANDS WITH THE DEVIL: THE FAILURE OF HUMANITY
TO ACT IN RWANDA, Arrow Books, London.

   Gourevitch, P 1998, WE WISH TO INFORM YOU THAT TOMORROW WE WILL BE
KILLED WITH OUR FAMILIES: STORIES FROM RWANDA, Farrar, Straus and Giroux, New
York.

   Melvern, L 2004, op cit. For a brief overview of Rwanda's History, we used: Booth, J and Briggs
P 2006, RWANDA, Bradt Travel Guides Ltd., Bucks.

When Charles, my guide, began to cry and I along with him, he explained that he was one of only seven survivors. He had hidden under a dead, blood-soaked older man until finally, one night, driven by thirst he had crawled away to hide in a swamp. Charles showed me the skull of his 'protector', complete with the machete mark. It was there, lined up in the crypt along with thousands of others. His clothes were among the piles I had seen on arrival. It is hard now to believe the horror that swept across this land in 1994 but, for Charles, it was a reality he lived, day after day. I was to hear similar stories to his, again and again.

Was hate now frozen in Rwanda? Had the population forgotten and forgiven their way to recovery or did retribution smoulder in the hearts of members of both communities? Had the cycle been broken? I didn't know, but from my limited observation the remedial action needing to be taken seemed twofold. First, bring justice and then close the wound. Second, change the attitudes of the emerging younger generation, primarily through education but also through government leadership. Outwardly, when I arrived, Rwanda seemed to have done a remarkable job of healing its wounds. Certainly it had achieved an astonishing level of economic growth and security. But with almost 84% of the population living in rural areas, it was difficult to know what people were really thinking. It was presumed that tensions must still exist with the Hutu outnumbering the Tutsi by more than four to one. Nonetheless, considering the inherent problems faced by almost all countries in sub-Saharan Africa, even without the aftermath of genocide, I saw the achievements of the past fifteen years as extraordinary. It would have been all too easy for Kagame's army to have embarked on a campaign of revenge and reprisal. They didn't, although ongoing military actions in Zaire, now renamed the Congo, have been continually questioned. To me, in 2010, the future of the country was being shaped by the following realities: half the cabinet was Hutu; more was spent on education than defence; it was East Africa's number one IT nation; and more than 54% of the National Assembly were women, the highest for any country in the world.[13] When questioned on why the country was making so much progress, a representative of the Rwandan National Commission for Human Rights explained to me that this was what happened "when you have been sick for so long and you realise you're still alive, and then when you have a President as the doctor, you stand up and start to recover". In short, it took political strength, something which Paul Kagame seemed to have in abundance.

---

[13]As of January 1, 2017, Rwanda's Lower House comprised 61.3% women, and the Upper House 38.5%, still the highest for any country. Source: Inter-Parliamentary Union 2017, *Women in National Parliaments*, http://www.ipu.org/wmn-e/classif.htm.

From the perspective of UNFPA, where his government had succeeded was in the area of family planning:

> Between 2000 and 2014 [through a combination of political will, community mobilization and rebuilding the health system], the country's Public-sector Family Planning Programme Impact Score (PFPI) grew from 8% to 57%, the most rapid rise in any African country. In addition, Rwanda's modern Contraceptive Prevalence Rate (mCPR) increased from 4% to 45% between 2000 and 2010, leading to its family planning programme being hailed as a phenomenal success.[14]

My first encounter with the President came soon after my arrival when I heard him speak to a group of young international students. The event was a gala ceremony at a big international hotel for the *Imbuto Foundation*, an NGO headed by the First Lady and aimed at supporting 'young Rwandan achievers'. When Kagame entered I saw that he was a very tall, very thin man. On this occasion he was dressed casually and, although he had prepared notes, spoke directly to the students. He told them in a slow and intense way how

> You cannot rely on anybody other than yourself. If you are poor and you do nothing, you will stay poor. If you work hard, you may not have time to sleep but you will achieve something. So, it is with our country. No one is ultimately going to save us just as no one, ultimately, is going to determine our fate; not the Europeans, the US, the UN or the Chinese. We are Rwandans. It is up to us just as it is up to you.

Kagame continued in the same vein. International aid, he said, was useful only to assist a country stand on its own feet, to enable countries that received aid to move on to become donors. "Independence, not dependence" is what he wanted for Rwanda—"if it is the latter, your dignity is eroded".[15] Simplistic but effective, I thought. After the President was photographed with the students, arms around them, I couldn't help comparing Kagame with those other cunning, corrupt, and long-serving African leaders. I set out to find more about him.

---

[14]Bongaarts, J and Hardee, K 2017, *'The Role of Public-Sector Family Planning Programs in Meeting the Demand for Contraception in Sub-Saharan Africa'*, vol. 43, no. 2.

[15]President Kagame in response to being questioned on whether Africa needed more investment than international aid, at the International Leadership Programme: A Global Intergenerational Forum in Kigali Rwanda, January 1–9, 2010.

I was told he does not live ostentatiously, nor did I see or hear any evidence that either he or his family was corrupt. I was surprised to see that his photo was not located in every classroom or government office as some other national leaders required. I was never held up in traffic waiting for one of those endless presidential motorcades to pass by, as was repeatedly the case in Kenya. I was told that when Kagame says something, ministers either act upon it or were dismissed. Unlike my experience in Bangladesh I was informed his government did not pilot projects, but if initiatives worked in other countries they would try it.

To me, Kagame's unique approach was no more evident than in the practice of *Umuganda* as explained by our office driver when I first arrived. This monthly event was the modern equivalent of a traditional Rwandan practice whereby you assisted your neighbours—by building their house or cultivating their fields or generally being supportive and doing it all for free. The observance now was also intended to encourage people to think nationally, not ethnically, something many could not have imagined a few years previously. In the same vein, I was told how he interviewed local administrators on television once a year and required them to explain their progress during the previous 12 months. Failure to deliver could mean the end of a career. He was said not to shy away from being questioned himself and senior bureaucrats were encouraged to do so. Kagame had certainly brought unity and stability, and people admired him for that. But I had no doubt he was ruthless.

Because of the genocide, supporters of Kagame told me that Rwanda was a 'special case'. The government took a hard line on dissent, they said, out of concern that those ethnic tensions which ignited the atrocities, should not be allowed to resurface. In the view of many, the democracy practised by the west was still not relevant, nor were criticisms from those who had never experienced such horrors. As long as Rwandans understood this thinking, Kagame maintained, they wanted to move on.[16]

During my time in Kigali I attended everything I could. My aim was to immerse myself in the country and its culture. Because of the genocide and its aftermath, it was all very compelling. I repeatedly asked questions as I tried to piece together a portrait of this place. I realised that my natural interest in people, events, politics and history, plus a willingness to engage and then the patience to listen, helped me at such times. When I first met the Rwandans they said very little. Was it language or self-protection or shyness? Later, I discovered that if I smiled and chatted on then there was an immediate change, faces lit up and you had an exchange. I spent a lot of time with my

---

[16] Ibid.

colleagues. I made a commitment to visit each of them at home and meet with their families. Because I knew they all went to church, it was assumed I would go as well. Where better to begin that home visit than by first joining them in their weekly worship. Not only did I enjoy these interactions, build friendships and collegiality but I listened and learnt.

My starting point was the Catholic cathedral in Kigali. It was not a cathedral in the grand European sense. It resembled more a warehouse. A large, octagonal building, open at the sides, it consisted of a tiered concrete floor, row after row of shabby plastic seating and, at the front, an altar flanked by cheap Catholic icons (a white Virgin Mary gazing down with arms outspread, a Jesus on the cross and a heroic saint, Saint George, spearing a dragon). What made the service memorable was the choir. Forty red-robed men and women swaying back and forth as they sang and clapped their way through hymns and responses. The priest was in white, trimmed with green, as were the altar boys. Incense was burned, communion was taken, and the sermon delivered in English. I clapped, joined in, and tried to follow. Later, I ate lunch with the family of the staff member who had invited me to church. They lived in a basic, single-story, concrete slab construction adjacent to a new three-storied home in the process of being built. We sat on the concrete foundations and, along with various family members who seemed to drift in, had a typical Rwandese lunch—sweet potato, beans, cassava and corn (*isombe*), peas, millet, chicken (being city folk they ate meat which was often not the case in rural areas) and fried plantains (*mizuzu*).

Another Sunday saw me attending the 10 o'clock service at the 'Evangelical Restoration' church in Kinyarwanda. This time I was with our office receptionist. She was born in Kinshasa, Zaire, of Rwandese parents but, like many others, was forced to relocate to Rwanda following expulsion from that country. She was dressed in her Sunday finery: full-length colourful dress, the wrap around head scarf with bag and makeup to match. French was her first language. Gracious and generous in manner, she had been a 'born-again' since the age of 12.

The church was built after the genocide. It was more solid than the cathedral and, in keeping with its evangelical tradition, had no adornments (no crosses, altars, pictures etc). It was a much bigger crowd than the Catholics the week before, although that also was a large one. Now, there were over a thousand in attendance. The service was an inspiration. It began when the choir of 40—led by a male singer out front, backed by six others just behind—opened the singing. They were accompanied by three guitarists, a drummer, and a keyboard player. Half an hour later we were all still singing, clapping, waving our hands back and forth and, periodically, jumping up and down like the Masai. Even the 40-odd dark-suited elders sitting with me in the front rows were moved by the spirit, any sense of reserve having left them. Once the singing had finished and the choir had filed off the stage—some to join the teenagers in the congregation, others the children on the mezzanine floor—the deputy pastor, dressed immaculately in a pinstriped suit, came forward to deliver the sermon. He had chosen the subject of planting seed, on the barren, the sandy and the fertile soil. His text consisted of eight passages taken from the Old and New Testaments. As he referred to each of these readings, many in the congregation followed in their own bibles, marking the passages, and taking notes of his explanations. He spoke of the quality of the seed, not just the soil in which it was planted. He asked questions of the congregation, who answered directly or with an "amen". Like any good speaker he had a beginning, a middle, and a summary at the end. He also moved about as he spoke. Walking across the stage and with arms outstretched, he reached out to those on the left, the right and then to those in the centre. At the end, people came forward to declare their commitment to Jesus and to be embraced by the pastor and the elders. What a two and a half hours! Was it like this before the genocide, I asked myself, or had this congregation formed as a retreat from that horror? When it was finally over and, to my disappointment, the singing had ended, we headed out to the car park. There we met others, chatted and then adjourned to my colleague's home, via her Ford pickup, for lunch. What a wonderful day it had been. I felt fortunate.

Drivers have always been important to me in all my postings. I came to appreciate their value and friendship from my very first assignment in Bangladesh. You spent a lot of time in their company. In Kigali I made a visit to the home of one of our drivers. Born in Uganda, he had come to Rwanda in the nineties looking for work. He again returned after the genocide, found a job with the UN and married a local. He was now the father of four children, aged from 12 down. To reach his home you had to leave one of the few paved roads and rock and bump your way down a dirt track, past the continuous pedestrian traffic, until you reached his house. There was no garden, just packed earth on all sides. Once inside you were in semi-darkness, often the case as the one fluorescent light was not strong enough to illuminate the whole room. The furniture was a couple of sofas, a dining table and chairs, a glassed-in cabinet with trophies, glasses and other knick-knacks. There was also a bookcase full of schoolbooks, carefully covered in brown paper. A portrait of Jesus hung on the wall. It looked down on a television covered in a white embroidered cloth. Unfortunately, the television did not work due to the irregular power supply. The kitchen, with its wood fire, was out the back.

It was a typical lower middle-class Kigali home. As we drank African tea and ate ground nuts, the 12-year-old son produced his green and white plastic computer. It was one of those $200 laptops pioneered by Professor Negroponte of MIT who had set out to manufacture a low-cost computer for use by children in developing countries. With donor support, the Rwandan government was distributing 100,000 of these to nine to twelve-year old school children.[17] It looked like a Fisher Price toy encased in its colourful plastic, but it performed the basic functions and the boy could demonstrate them all. In his slow, deliberate English you could hear how he was consuming knowledge. It was impressive. While he was showing me how his laptop worked, we were interrupted by the arrival of his grandmother. "She is a born-again preacher," he told me, "and because she doesn't speak English, I have translated all her sermons into English and saved them on my computer!". The grandmother then, with her grandson translating, carefully and slowly set out to determine whether I had been saved or not.

I was grateful for this company on a Sunday as it formed part of my coping mechanism for occupying those empty times on the weekends. Moreover, it sealed bonds with colleagues and, as I listened to their stories, helped me weave together the fabric of this extraordinary country. On the Saturdays when I was on my own, I read the international press, listened to the BBC, went to the gym, and then spent the afternoon in the office.

It was almost immediately after my arrival, that I attended my first aerobic class. As soccer is to my son when settling in a new place so aerobics is to me. Somewhere to meet, greet and feel healthy. The class was meant to start at 6 p.m. and as I stood there in the dark, I wondered what was to happen or not happen. "We start when the participants arrive", I was told, "so just go and work out on the machines". "Okay." I drifted into the equipment room and kept an eye out for the stragglers. I soon discovered that the classes never started on time and that, for me, was a problem. Not because they started five minutes late, ten minutes and sometimes fifteen minutes late but when I also started to show up late, I often found they had started without me! Not surprisingly, the class had a distinct African flavour. Firstly, there were lots of men attending unlike aerobic sessions I have attended elsewhere. Along with the women, they spanned all ages and sizes. Being big and heavy was no

---

[17]Rwanda had piloted a one laptop per child program and planned to distribute 100,000 more computers—at $181 each—to children by June 2011. A year after that, it wanted to distribute laptops to half of Rwanda's 2.5 million schoolchildren.

Wadhams, N 2010, 'Can One Laptop Per Child Transform Rwanda's Economy?', Time, http://content.time.com/time/world/article/0,8599,1997940,00.html.

For more on this project, see the One Laptop Per Child website, one.laptop.org.

obstacle, nor should it have been. Only the occasional junior staff member from the UN fulfilled the standard slim Western stereotype. The instructor was lively. He bounced around and regularly turned off the sound so he could hear all the participants counting the movements. When the music was something everyone knew people sang along and there was always lots of chatter and exclamations throughout the pauses for rest (unlike Australia where there is scarcely a murmur).

Later, I added another outing to my weekend routine. I found a restaurant, run by an American couple, ex-Peace Corps, where every Saturday night they would show a film. Along I would go, be shown to a table, take my meal and watch the movie. They were quite recent ones. In fact, I could see a film the same week as my wife saw it back at home. Locals and expats attended, the young volunteers sitting with the long-time residents. Sitting under an open sky, it reminded me of Rabaul, Papua New Guinea, more than thirty years earlier when I would watch the latest Hollywood import sitting on camp chairs under a star-filled night.[18]

As a diplomat, I was officially invited to formal government events in which I was happy to immerse myself. In February, I joined the corps at the Parliamentary building for the annual launch of the judicial year. We had to be there by 9 o'clock, the President being scheduled to arrive at 10:30. As I lined up to clear security, I couldn't help noticing the shell holes pockmarking the walls, a visible reminder of the fighting that took place in April 1994 as hundreds of Rwandan Patriotic Front soldiers (there, as part of the Arusha Peace Accord) sought refuge before escaping and re-joining Kagame's invading forces in the east. Neither cameras nor mobile phones were allowed in the Parliament. X-ray screening was mandatory as was a pat down by an official. This was my first time in the Chamber of Deputies and I was eager to see what it looked like. It was a tiered structure rather like a large concert hall. I couldn't tell where the members sat but there was an electronic scoreboard for recording votes. High on the wall above where the speaker sat was a photo of the President. This set me to reflect on the separation of powers. But I cast aside such incendiary thoughts once I observed the 'Members of the Superior Council of the Judiciary' seated on the official platform as they awaited the President. They were splendid in their cherry red robes with white trim and black pillbox hats, ringed by different colours to designate rank. It was explained to me that this was the traditional regalia worn by French and Belgian judges under the Napoleonic Code that the legal system in Rwanda followed. There were eight men and seven women judges, including the Chief

---

[18]I was again in Papua New Guinea in 2012 acting as the UNFPA Representative.

Justice, seated as members of the Council. Facing them were row after row of red or black robed lower-ranked justices and lawyers. At the back, well behind us, was the military band, and after the President entered—45 min late—and shook hands with the justices, they played the national anthem. We all stood. Speeches were made, reports presented, and then it was time for the President to speak. As usual, his remarks were interesting, although it was difficult to follow given poor translation. He began by asking why there was a separate rostrum just for him in the middle of the floor, when the Prosecutor General and the Chief Justice had spoken at another lectern away to the side. He recounted a biblical story about a man pursued by a lion, who rapidly climbed a tree to escape. After some time, he told us, the lion tired, went away and the man scampered down and raced home. When he arrived at his village, the people gathered round and asked him what had happened. "Before I tell you", he replied, "I have to pray to God for saving me from a lion". "Why pray to God," came the response, "better you pray to the lion!" The story brought much laughter. Everyone roared. As I had heard from Kagame before, the gist of his remarks and the telling of this story, had to do with being self-reliant. It was up to each Rwandan, he was saying, to better themselves. Don't depend on others. He was like a coach urging on his listeners on to achieve his vision. Although he had a folder in front of him, he was not reading but exhorting his audience to join him in moving the country forward along his chosen path.

What was also interesting was who was sitting next to me on that morning. On one side I had a UN colleague who had been in Rwanda for some time. She told me how the country had so transformed itself in the years she had been there, that it was scarcely recognisable. On the other side, was the representative of 'Lawyers without Borders'. I vaguely knew there was such an NGO but had never met anyone from it. He was French and had served in Afghanistan (where he said all hope had gone despite the defeat of the Taliban). He had also served in Iran (where his conclusion was that the religious authorities would fight to stay in power because they had nowhere else to go. As a consequence, he said, they had strung the West along with their 'nuclear weapons play'). When this lawyer's representative first came to Rwanda he worked for 'Prisons Reform International', monitoring and reporting on prison conditions. They were absolutely appalling, he said. He described how the system was starved of funds with prisoners living in grossly overcrowded conditions and dying of TB, AIDS and every other possible illness. Previously, families could supply food, but not anymore. Now that he was working for the lawyers, my neighbour told me of the increasing challenges lawyers faced in Rwanda: a "narrowing of openness and increased sensitivity to any criticism". He spoke of the approaching elections and how an opposition candidate was struggling to campaign and how pressure was being applied to two independent newspapers. I listened intently as he described the skilful way in which the Government countered its opposition and handled the probing questions coming from donors.

The "Lawyers without Borders" representative also told me of the '*Gacaca*', a system of local justice re-established after the genocide to deal with the enormous backlog of cases in its aftermath. Under this traditional system, villagers would gather together on a patch of grass to discuss issues and resolve conflicts between families, with heads of households acting as judges. With over 100,000 genocide suspects still in gaol after eight years (although figures as to the exact number varied considerably), it was estimated it would take 200–400 years for the normal judicial system to clear the backlog.[19] So, a decision was made to reinstitute this traditional form of dispensing justice. By 2001, 255,000 lay judges had been elected. They began hearing cases in June 2002.[20] In January 2010, I had the chance to attend this tribunal, and spent a day in a crowded schoolroom hearing the trials of six prisoners who were accused of killing their neighbours. It was held in a rural area, in a village, and we drove up to it in our four-wheel drive. When we arrived, there were quite a few people standing outside. They took some interest in our presence, but no one questioned why we were there. There were also a number of men milling together on the periphery. Dressed in simple orange pants and tops, these were the prisoners. I had regularly come across such groups when driving through the countryside. You saw them in their orange jumpsuits working in the fields with one sleepy guard keeping watch over them. You waved as you passed by and they would wave back. I was struck by the fact that these prisoners about to be tried had earlier lived in a village, had had the same neighbours for generations of whom some were in the court, yet during the three months of the genocide had committed unspeakable acts.

The *Gacaca* room was set up like a traditional court. It consisted of five judges, each wearing sashes signifying their rank. The room was packed. You could not have crowded any more people in. Some had even spilled outside.

---

[19]The UN Tribunal sitting in Arusha, Tanzania, had only 71 cases brought before it over a period of 20 years (1995–2015). Of this number, 62 people were sentenced, 14 acquitted, 10 referred to national jurisdictions for trial, 3 fugitives referred to the Mechanism for International Criminal Tribunals (MICT), 2 deceased before judgment and 2 indictments withdrawn before trial (*The ICTR in Brief*, United Nations Mechanism for International Criminal Tribunals, viewed 19 December 2017). The total estimated cost was US$2 billion (Leithead, A 2015, 'Rwanda Genocide: International Criminal Tribunal Closes', *BBC News, 14 December.*

[20]These figures are cited on page 356 of Daly, E 2002, 'Between Punitive and Reconstructive Justice: The Gacaca Courts in Rwanda', *New York University Journal of International Law and Politics,* vol. 34, no. 2, 355–396.

They seated us up the front. I sat beside a national colleague who whispered translations from the Rwandese into my ear. We began with a moment of silence and then the president of the court explained the procedural instructions including how to behave. You could be thrown out and put in gaol for violating these, he said. We were in session. The judge read out the allegations against the first prisoner and ran through the events of what had allegedly happened. He then opened the floor for anyone to speak. People stood and recounted what they recalled and ended by demanding the prisoner answer why he did it, who organised the killings and what he and the others did with the bodies. Some of the accused were as young as thirteen at the time of the killings. The prisoners were able to respond, and there were long exchanges. One woman, whose sister had been killed, declared she had no confidence in the hearings as she did not trust this "corrupted" court. Back and forth it went with witnesses accusing, pointing fingers, questioning, demanding justice and the accused repeatedly denying, claiming they were not there and calling for information earlier presented to be reintroduced.

There were six cases heard on that day. As they proceeded, the weather grew hotter. To avoid disruption, my translator and I leaned as far forward as we could with elbows on knees and the sweat dripping off us. The proceedings continued into the evening until the presiding judge called for a halt and rescheduled the court to sit another day. I never did hear the outcome. My sense from this very limited experience was that given the number of outstanding cases plus the duration of time prisoners were spending in jail without their cases being heard, the government had little alternative but to proceed. It was very questionable justice but hundreds of thousands of cases were heard. The backlog was cleared with 86% of those who went through the system, according to the Rwandan government, being found guilty.[21] There were unexpected consequences, however, with prominent Rwandans being accused and having to defend themselves. Critics saw the whole exercise as a form of mass justice whereby the Hutu population were collectively found guilty. It was victor's justice, they claimed.

The aftermath of the genocide was in many ways as catastrophic as the horrors of 1994. I saw evidence of this when I visited a refugee camp near the Congo border on the edge of Lake Kivu, in the Rubavu district. To get there you drove through hilly countryside, intensively cultivated, and divided by gullies smelling of those Australian eucalypts. At the camp a UNHCR volunteer welcomed me. She told me there had been three camps in the country since 1996 and that currently there were 53,000 Congolese refugees in one of

---

[21]Government sources put the number of those found guilty at 86% out of the 1,958,634 cases heard (Rwandapedia, 'Gacaca', http://www.rwandapedia.rw/explore/gacaca.

them. They were mostly semi-literate farmers, she said, who had nowhere to go. Most were women—the men stayed to fight. All had escaped the conflict, plus the disease and the raping. My team and I had come to distribute thousands of hygiene kits to these women, kits which I had arranged to be trucked up from Kenya.

Like other refugee camps I had visited, the one in the Rubavu district for Congolese was a wretched place. Located near the town of Gisenyi, it was opposite Goma on the other side of the border. Unlike the surrounding valleys, this camp sat on volcanic rock. It was cold, windswept, and desolate. 18,000 people were housed in tents made of plastic. There were no floors. The toilets were few. They overflowed. People cooked for themselves on basic facilities located in rusted shipping containers. There were few means of earning an income. The Jesuits ran the schools, but there were not enough. The youth were desperate for an upper secondary school. There was nothing for them or anybody else to do but wait and hope the situation in the Congo would improve, so they could return home. Most had been waiting for years. They were living a miserable life.

The other two camps I worked in were for Rwandan refugees from the genocide who had been hiding in the eastern Congo since 1994. During 2009, 20,000 had made the trek back home and crossed the border. They arrived with nothing but were met and then bussed to a camp inside Rwanda where they were given ID cards, medical insurance, a map, plastic sheets, hoes, kitchen sets and three months' supply of food. They were also briefed on the changes that had occurred since 1994 such as the new structure of Rwanda and the different place names that had been given. After spending two or three days in the camps, they were expected to return to the homes from which they had fled.

While these people waited, life continued around them. Soon after my arrival, I attended a donor meeting at the Lake Kivu Serena Hotel. Located on the outskirts of Gisenyi it sent its guests off to sleep at night with the invocation to "*Lala salama*", meaning sleep well in Swahili. I wondered, as I settled down in my bed, how many during the preceding decade and a half had slept soundly as war raged just within walking distance of my room. Still, I couldn't help being struck with the exotic ring to the location where this meeting took place. International hotels like this can be like any other, be they in Thailand or Kenya or wherever, but this one was right in the centre of Africa. It was located on a beach fronting a lake where volcanic vents powered the adjacent towns. Close by were the gorillas, "in the mist", made famous by Dian Fossey. Who built such a hotel, I asked myself, and why here? Then again, why shouldn't it be here? Why shouldn't a beautiful lake have a tourist hotel on its foreshore? But not so long ago there had been a war and even now there was military activity just across the border.

I was reminded of this fragility, as I stepped out of my car on arrival, and was greeted by an American Marine captain. Advancing across the driveway, hand outstretched, he told me his name was Chuck. "Come on in", he gestured, "Where are you from?" I was more eager to ask him that question and find out what he was doing here. Chuck had no hesitation in telling me, explaining that he was here to train Rwandan troops, stationed up in the nearby hills, who may or not have been making incursions across the border. As he talked, I was impressed. Chuck showed a detailed command of his assignment. Later, as we walked into lunch, he was warmly welcomed by another soldier. This time it was a UN military peace-keeping officer, in charge of a contingent of resident Uruguayan troops. As I sat between these two officers, sipping my soup, I was struck by the incongruity of one charged with keeping the peace, the other preparing to challenge it and my having to deal with the consequences.

Meanwhile, back in Kigali, the routine work of UNFPA continued. As I was there as a trouble shooter, it was expected I would focus on the office. From one-on-one interviews with the staff, I learnt that the previous representative had been transferred following a two-year stint marked by rising tension and division. An illustration of this came when I enquired about the administrative budget, seeking funds to mend broken blinds and reduce the sun pouring in which both blinded and heated you at the same time. This did not just occur in my office but along the entire west side of the building. To escape the glare, the staff had resorted to pasting paper over the glass. I determined to do something about it. But when I enquired about the necessary finance, I was told there were no funds left. Where had they gone? To sound-proofing the representative's office, I was told. $2,500 had been spent to insulate the doors because she suspected the staff was listening to her conversations. So much for cohesion and team building. Then, it came to light, that not only were the national staff not trusted, they were further alienated when the Representative chose only to speak to her favourites who were the young foreign volunteers (putting them into an untenable situation). Ignoring local professionals for outsiders was never a good recipe for collaborative endeavour, especially, in a climate where ethnic divisions had had such disastrous consequences. I ignored the soundproofing and never closed my door. I never have in all my assignments. I don't like closed doors, nor do I think it's good practice, suggestive as it is of a confidential agenda which runs counter to being open to staff and walking out to see them. Besides, I was told the soundproofing didn't work.

I was given more snippets of office life as I came to know my colleagues. One told me, as we walked together across the road to buy a sandwich, that a previous representative had never walked anywhere, even next door. They expected the driver to deliver them, flag flying. Another told me of being lectured on how inappropriate it was that the representative had to carry their own bag at a public event. That was for a junior to do! Not surprisingly, these hierarchical divisions led to a culture of distrust, where staff were unwilling to interact and share information for fear of reprisal. I was reminded again of what I had seen many times before when Chief of Human Resources. Gossip and rumour becoming the norms of office life with each staff member assessing themselves on their interaction with the representative and not programme performance.

When hearing these stories, I wondered what had happened to all those managerial and team-building competencies UNFPA supposedly tested for before appointing a representative. Were they a sham? Perhaps they weren't applied in all cases. As I well knew, political and personal appointments did happen. Representatives also had different views of their role and their status. Certainly, in Rwanda's case, I was only hearing one side of the story. Nonetheless, there was a crisis. But in classic UN practice, the staff member(s) had simply been moved on, never told of their shortcomings, and left convinced of their own legitimacy. As seen earlier during my years in New York, such behaviour was typical of a type of leadership not uncommon in the UN system. My troubleshooting in Rwanda brought home to me that in an organisation like UNFPA, good leadership and management were essential to the effective running of both country offices and the wider UN system.

I later saw how divisive attitudes were not just confined to the odd UN office. At a meeting of the donor community, it was the Belgian representative who continually interjected, commented, joked, walked around and dominated proceedings. He was tolerated, even laughed at albeit in a grim way. We should have told him to sit down and be quiet but we didn't. Diplomatic niceties prevailed. Later, one of my African colleagues said the Belgian was well known for this behaviour, which the colleague rightly described as colonialist.

But here in Kigali it was now my turn to right perceived wrongs. I was expected to meld the office into a more professional, structured, and focused unit. All that time spent getting to know the staff, listening to them, understanding their assignments, scrutinising the environment, and comprehending the challenges, had to lead to some transformation. What was it going to be? How to build on the successes and address the weaknesses?

I opted for a one-week retreat on team building to be held in Gisenyi. The objectives were to discuss what makes an effective team; to understand team styles and culture; to develop conflict and communication management approaches; to understand effective leadership; and to set goals for the year ahead. Activities would include everything from social outings to classroom-based work, problem-solving activities and crisis-handling sessions. The main facilitator came from a consulting firm in Johannesburg. He began by interviewing staff, preparing personal profiles, and then using these to construct formulas for effective team building. He spoke English and French. What an asset this language ability was for successful interactive sessions; the capacity to move between languages with ease just like those bus drivers first heard by me when arriving in Geneva back in the seventies. Now, our staff were analysing those attitudes underlaying their behaviour and looking at ways to translate strategy into measurable action. We discussed positive and negative ways to acknowledge colleagues, how to use time, how to communicate, how to be accountable and how to be respectful and behave with integrity. Finally, we looked at the changes that were taking place in the office, likely reactions to them, and suggestions for how to remain positive. Did it work? Well, training makes no sense if afterwards things revert back to the status quo. Lessons learnt have to be implemented and follow-up tasks completed. We had to have an action plan with measurable goals. That was developed. Its recommendations were implemented and are now reviewed on a semestral basis at further office retreats.[22]

Aside from these staffing issues, there were also programme issues to be addressed. First, I needed to find out what we were actually doing and with what results. Whilst this may not sound difficult, when you add in the UN's obsession with development jargon, to know exactly what we were doing, whether or not we had achieved our goals and whether we could see a connection between these and the objectives of the country programme, was a challenge. First, to sort through the jargon. Again and again references were made to "incentivisation, deliverables, concretise, tracer sector, functionality, modalities, harmonisation, alignment, benchmarks, operationalize, pooled funding, management instruments, utilisation, roadmaps" and, of course, everything was "integrated and proactive". Then, there were all the acronyms.

As I had observed elsewhere, the programme in Rwanda was too diffuse, consisting of too many disparate activities. This made it difficult to monitor,

---

[22]As informed by a colleague based in Kigali in recent years.

let alone evaluate. In my view, it was better to make a measurable difference in fewer districts than spend time processing limited amounts of money
across many. With a small office we needed to focus on strategic outcomes, on
having an impact on government, rather than being encumbered by procedural necessities. What was happening was that administrative inputs were
trumping project outcomes. 'Moving the files' had become the mantra of
middle management and when there were not enough managers to complete
this task (or they were unwilling to do it), there was an over-reliance on JPOs
and UNV's. As a result, they were seen as just another staff member and not a
young trainee requiring mentoring and exposure across a range of experiences.

But UNFPA Rwanda was not alone in its struggles to strategically priori-
tise. WHO had even more projects covering amounts big and small. Likewise,
UNICEF. Then there were the multiple small agencies which after adding
in the big four—UNDP, UNICEF, WHO and UNFPA—totalled 22 UN
offices operating in Rwanda.[23] How could each of these effectively monitor
and evaluate let alone engage in policy dialogue? How could any Minister
of Health and their staff, for example, keep up with the representations
made by agencies, multilateral and bilateral, each pushing their own agendas
covering different time frames and financial commitments? They were unable
to. Duplication and competition were inevitable. Bring on UN reform, I said.

The good news in Kigali was that reform was already under way. Before
I arrived, I was heartened to read that Rwanda was one of eight coun-
tries that volunteered to pilot the 'Delivering as One' (DaO) initiative.[24] It
was being implemented under the United Nations Development Assistance
Framework (UNDAF), which was aligned with the Rwandan government's
"Economic Development and Poverty Reduction Strategy" and the "Rwanda
Vision 2020".

When I looked at the paperwork on reform it looked good. Lots of attractive folders and substantial documentation. The objective was to "improve the
impact, coherence, efficiency and positioning of the UN system in Rwanda"
to enable it to better help the country meet the MDGs. [25] But given
my fixation on measuring "impact", I couldn't help asking what level of
"improvement" was sought? What was the status right now, I enquired, and
how would you know when it was "improved"? In fact, were those measurable

---

[23] For more on the agencies that operate in Rwanda, see the One UN Rwanda site: http://www.rw.
one.un.org/who-we-are/un-agencies-rwanda.

[24] For more on Delivering as One, see the independent country led evaluation.
   Universalia Management Group 2010, *Country Led Evaluation of Delivering as One in Rwanda:
Final Report*.

[25] Page 3 of Universalia Management Group Report, ibid.

"efficiencies" earmarked? And against whom was the UN seeking to "position" itself? Was it USAID, the World Bank, or the European Union? Within our own system, could one agency accept that another was more competent than it to deliver a UN development goal? Could we divide the country into spheres of influence or allocate specific sectors to the most resourceful agency? And, as a consequence, would transaction costs be reduced? Or, given the all-encompassing wants of the UN family of agencies, funds and programmes, did each one of them still want to be part of the action, real or imagined, with none seeing themselves phasing out to national execution? In short, what was "Delivering as One" actually achieving? Was it still the old UN chestnut that "when all's said and done, more would be said than done"?

The answer came following an independent review, undertaken in 2010, which found that the "One UN seemed far more rhetorical than substantive; (that it was) known only to a small group of UN staff, government workers and NGOs. Those who worked closely with the UN knew the agency they worked with, not the One UN system".[26] Briefly stated, "One UN" seemed a good idea in principle but was just not all there in practice. Later, much later, despite this awkward beginning, I heard that the UN Team was making progress. Theme groups were functioning and proving effective. There was enhanced cooperation among agencies resulting in reduced duplication. Joint planning and sharing of duties were said to be leading to improved efficiency. Pleasingly, UNFPA had become a leader and the combined UN presence was seen as adapting to Rwanda's changing priorities and needs. Despite this encouraging report, I still felt it was too early to evaluate the long-term impact of the reform initiative. As I had seen earlier, the UN practice of detailing results in the most convoluted way intended to please everybody and annoy none, made forecasting the future an exercise requiring extreme patience. Add to this the reality that everything undertaken in Rwanda is done at the behest of the government. It is the government under the leadership of President Kagame, and not the "Delivering as One" initiative nor the wider UN system, that dictates the necessity for and actions of the UN in Rwanda. That 2010 report found that if the government needed to turn to a specific agency, it did so, irrespective of the "Delivering as One" initiative. It was largely irrelevant. Of course, the environment in which the UN operates could change, if Kagame wanted it to, but based upon my interaction with him and the views he expressed over the failings of the UN in the past, I think this is unlikely. I suspect the development work of the UN is largely a sideshow to his national

---

[26]ibid

agenda, except where it gives him a global platform to proclaim his country's successes.[27] Foreign aid may be 30 per cent to 40 per cent of Rwanda's budget currently[28] but of that amount the actual total coming from the UN system, as distinct from the all-in budgeted wish-list, is relatively minor.

As I write these words, I am again troubled by the realisation that I am criticising my own organisation and the UN creed about which I am passionate. I am loath to do so. Despite its failings, of which there are many, the norm in my working life and that of my UN colleagues has been one of commitment, endeavour, and harmony. In Rwanda, we all worked collegially in what had been in the nineties one of the most difficult environments imaginable. In spite of the apparent differences in origin, culture, religion and language, there was a universality in the workplace that bound us together as UN staff. This was illustrated for me on the last night of our staff retreat. We were on the banks of Lake Kivu looking across at the Eastern Congo. All the UN staff were there. They were mostly Rwandese but included Senegalese, Cameroonians, Norwegians, Dutch, Serbs, and Congolese. At the end of our retreat we decided to have a barbeque. People produced various items of food, a grill was found, and wood was collected. To begin with we had a game of volleyball on the sand and then we enjoyed a wonderful meal. After it was over, out came the guitars and the drums and we proceeded to sing and dance the night away. Despite the wide variation in backgrounds and the exhaustion, there was a feeling of unity in our coming together. Out there, in the middle of Africa, we were trying to make a difference. That was what my work for the UN was all about.

---

[27] "At the 2012 London Summit on Family Planning, President Paul Kagame expressed his vision for Rwanda to become a middle-income country in the context of equipping women and men to plan their families" Bongaarts and Hardee op cit.

[28] According to the World Bank's country overview on Rwanda, http://www.worldbank.org/en/country/rwanda/overview.

Index

Professor Howie is currently writing a book on the UN's efforts to reform its development role.

© The Editor(s) (if applicable) and The Author(s), under exclusive license to Springer Nature Switzerland AG 2021
I. Howie, *Reflections on a United Nations' Career*, Springer Biographies,
https://doi.org/10.1007/978-3-030-77063-1

CPSIA information can be obtained
at www.ICGtesting.com
Printed in the USA
LVHW080748041021
699441LV00002B/41

9 783030 770624